Handbook of ENT

Diseases and Disorders of the Ear, Nose, and Throat

CAJ Prescott

Cape Town
OXFORD UNIVERSITY PRESS
SOUTHERN AFRICA
1998

Oxford University Press
Great Clarendon Street, Oxford OX2 6DP, United Kingdom

offices in

Oxford New York
Auckland Bangkok Buenos Aires Cape Town Chennai
Dar es Salaam Delhi Hong Kong Istanbul Karachi Kolkata
Kuala Lumpur Madrid Melbourne Mexico City Mumbai Nairobi
São Paulo Shanghai Singapore Taipei Tokyo Toronto

Handbook of ENT: Diseases and Disorders of the Ear, Nose, and Throat

ISBN 0 19 571585 3

First Published 1998
Reprinted 2002

COPY EDITOR: Ethné Clarke
DESIGNER: Mark Standley
INDEXER: Jeanne Cope

Published by Oxford University Press Southern Africa,
PO Box 12119, N1 City, 7463, Cape Town, South Africa

Set in Utopia by RHT desktop publishing cc
Printed and bound by ABC Book Printers,
Kinghall Avenue, Epping Industria II

Every effort has been made to check drug dosages in this book. However, dosages continue to be revised and new side-effects recognized. Please consult the manufacturers' instructions before prescribing or administering the drugs mentioned here. The author and publishers cannot be held responsible for the misuse or misapplication of any drug information in this book.

Contents

Acknowledgements

The following comment was passed on to me while I was preparing this textbook: Isaac Newton, when complimented on his achievements, noted that they had only been possible because he was 'standing on the shoulders of giants'. This was particularly apt because, on reading my manuscript, I realized that I had incorporated ideas, words, and phrases from many 'giants' in this speciality which had, consciously and subconsciously, become part of my philosophy and approach. I apologize for the lack of specific references to these sources and trust that anyone reading this book who feels that what has been incorporated originated from them, will accept that this book is an attempt to build a framework of basic knowledge and skills that we, as teachers, need to pass on to future generations of clinicians in the same way that it was passed on to us, in order that their practice of our speciality is of an acceptable standard. There are, however, two people whose contributions require acknowledgement. The first is John Duff, my predecessor in charge of organizing our undergraduate ENT course at the University of Cape Town Medical School, whose notes form the basis for the chapters on anatomy and physiology. The second is Marie-Louise du Plessis, who prepared the original line drawings used to complement the text.

CAJ PRESCOTT
University of Cape Town

Introduction

Disorders of the ears, nose, and throat are commonly encountered in primary health care. It is estimated that between 20 and 30 per cent of patients seen in a typical practice present with these disorders. Some examples will serve to support this estimate:

- Almost all patients in a practice will have the occasional cold, which will frequently be followed by a period of purulent nasal discharge. Sometimes this will precipitate an attack of sinusitis.
- More than half of the children in any population will have an episode of acute otitis media before they start school – the peak incidence is in the one- to three-year age group – and many of these children will have had more than one episode by this age.
- We all produce wax in our ears. Some patients become preoccupied with removing this wax and persistently fiddle in their ears. At some stage, such fiddling either impacts the wax in the ear canal or precipitates an episode of otitis externa, particularly in warm, moist climates or in patients who often go swimming.
- Deafness is a particularly disabling problem, and hearing loss is one of the inevitable accompaniments of ageing that adds to the burdens of these 'golden' years. Recognition of the problem and direction towards assistance, usually in the form of hearing aids, can do much to ease the problem. Age is not the only cause of deafness, and, given some knowledge of the causes such as rubella in pregnancy and noise in industry, many are potentially preventable. Counselling in this regard is an essential part of the work of a primary care physician.
- Smokers invariably ignore health warnings and some smokers in any practice are likely to develop cancer. Although not as common as cancer in the lung, cancer in

the upper aerodigestive tract is sometimes encountered, particularly involving the tongue and the larynx. Early recognition may be life-saving. Treated Stage 1 laryngeal cancer patients have a 90 per cent five-year survival rate, whereas when the cancer has progressed to Stage 4, the survival rate falls below 50 per cent.

Despite all these factors, in most undergraduate medical courses, ENT is regarded as a minor speciality and is squeezed into one of the busy clinical years as a short course. For ENT tutors this poses the problem (and responsibility!) of how, in the short time available, to equip medical students with sufficient essential information and skills to enable them to recognize ENT disorders and to manage patients presenting with these disorders once they have graduated and have their own practices.

Aims

Tertiary education theory maintains that the first step to achieve this goal is to establish aims for the course.

Most students will have forgotten much of the anatomy and physiology they so painfully acquired in the early years of the medical course, so the first aim will be:

- **To refresh knowledge of essential ENT anatomy and physiology so that the 'normal' can be recognized.**

Eliciting essential signs in this area of multiple body orifices requires special examination skills. In the short time available, these skills can be acquired only if they are taught in a rigid, structured manner. Therefore the second aim will be:

- **To teach a structured approach to examination of the ear, the nose, the throat, and the head and neck region.**

The range of disorders encountered in ENT specialist practice is vast. Although many of these disorders require specialized knowledge and sophisticated diagnostic and management skills, most of them are common in a primary care practice and can be adequately managed in this setting.

Therefore the third aim will be:

- **To present students with an essential core knowledge of ENT disorders.**

Patients, however, do not present with disorders but with symptoms and signs which must be elicited to make the diagnosis of a disorder. Therefore the fourth aim will be:

- **To present a practical approach to ENT disorders.**

Some patients will present with disorders that will not be within the management competence of a primary care physician. Early recognition of those disorders requiring referral to a specialist service may be vital to the ultimate prognosis. Therefore the fifth aim will be:

- **To establish guidelines for specialist referral in ENT disorders. In this text, situations calling for referral are flagged with this symbol: R**

Patients have the right to expect that their primary care physician is competent to care for them. Therefore the sixth aim will be:

- **To assess the competence of students regarding their core knowledge, examination skills, and ability to diagnose and manage common ENT disorders.**

The community requires the services of physicians with above average knowledge and skills for the management of specialized ENT disorders. Therefore the final aim will be:

- **To stimulate in some students the desire to further pursue ENT through electives, research projects, further training, or specialist training.**

Objectives

Education theory further states that aims are achieved by setting objectives. Ideally, these objectives should be formulated in such a way that they act as stepping stones along the way to achieving each aim. However, in practice, most ENT departments have a busy clinical workload and are understaffed for teaching. For this reason it is almost impossible to set out objectives in a logical sequence when the theoretical teaching sessions have to be interspersed with clinical exposure. Whereas theory sessions can conveniently divide the speciality into its components – ear, nose, throat, head and neck – in the clinical sessions patients are going to present with disorders not yet covered by the theory. In practice, therefore, objectives have to be stated as set out below:

By the end of the ENT course students will:

- Have refreshed their knowledge of the essential anatomy and physiology of the ear, the nose, the throat, and the head and neck.
- Be aware of symptoms resulting from disorders of the ear, the nose, the throat, and the head and neck.
- Be able to examine the ear, the nose, the throat, and the head and neck; differentiate normal from abnormal; and recognize the nature of any abnormality.
- Be able to relate these symptoms and examination findings to an essential core knowledge of disorders of the ear, the nose, the throat, and the head and neck.
- Be able to initiate management for these disorders, and to set in motion the following:
  - procedures required to examine the area further
  - investigations required to confirm the diagnosis
  - primary care treatment of the disorder
  - follow-up care for the disorder
  - referral of patients when their disorders require specialist attention
  - undertaking of interim care while awaiting referral.

Assessment

According to education theory, these objectives should establish the criteria for assessment. To be most effective, assessment should be 'formative', that is, undertaken throughout the course to afford opportunities for the correction of deficiencies. However, for the reasons stated above, this is often impractical in busy ENT departments so that, for the most part, all that will be offered is 'summative' assessment, that is, assessment undertaken at the end of the course when it is usually too late to correct deficiencies except by repeating the course – the ever-present threat of failing the ENT examination!

An attempt has been made in this textbook to condense the knowledge, which an ENT surgeon will take several years of training and practice to acquire, into an essential core knowledge of theory and skills that can be imparted in a brief ENT undergraduate course to equip students as future medical graduates with sufficient basic ENT information to enable them to manage these disorders when encountered in primary care. It is strongly recommended that students add to the information contained in this book by referring to the many ENT textbooks available either in medical libraries or in medical bookshops in order to acquire a broader understanding of the different approaches to and ways of treating ENT disorders.

Students who are contemplating the purchase of another textbook to supplement this core knowledge manual should be aware of two considerations, apart from cost, that should influence their choice. The first consideration is the way they prefer to learn from a textbook. ENT books vary in both their style of presentation and in the amount of illustration. Some adopt the traditional style of presenting theoretical discussion of disorders by regions. Others adopt a more practical, symptom-oriented approach. Most fall somewhere between these and vary in the amount and quality of illustration. The second consideration is that some of these textbooks will really only be useful to undergraduates, whereas others will act as a reference source that will sustain them in primary care practice. Students would be best advised to consider these two aspects and then browse through what is available in the library before making their choice.

The 'ENT Ten'

If you learn nothing else from your ENT course, you should try to memorize these ten points and keep them in your memory bank for the rest of your career.

1. If a mother says her baby is deaf she is usually right.
2. A foul or unilateral nasal discharge in a child is usually due to a foreign body. In an adult suspect tumour.
3. An inflamed, swollen cheek is usually due to dental infection.
4. A painful, swollen eye may be caused by frontal or ethmoidal sinusitis. When this occurs, vision is at risk and there is potential for intracranial spread of infection.
5. Check for ear disease in all cases of meningitis and facial nerve palsy. When ear disease causes facial palsy, exclude TB.
6. If hoarseness persists for more than a month, entertain a suspicion of a tumour (cancer in smokers!) and refer urgently for a diagnosis to be made.
7. Pain referred to one ear is a sinister symptom in anyone over forty with a sore throat. Suspect malignancy!
8. Any neck swelling needs careful ENT evaluation prior to any invasive procedures.
9. Deafness in the elderly can be helped. Refer these patients for assessment.
10. People wanting to poke anything into their ears should use their elbow! Use syringing to remove wax, foreign bodies, and purulent discharges.

PART I
The ear

1 Structure and function of the ear

ENT surgeons describe the ear in three parts: the external, the middle, and the inner ear.

The external ear

The external ear consists of the pinna (auricle), the external auditory canal (external ear canal or simply ear canal), and the tympanic membrane (eardrum).

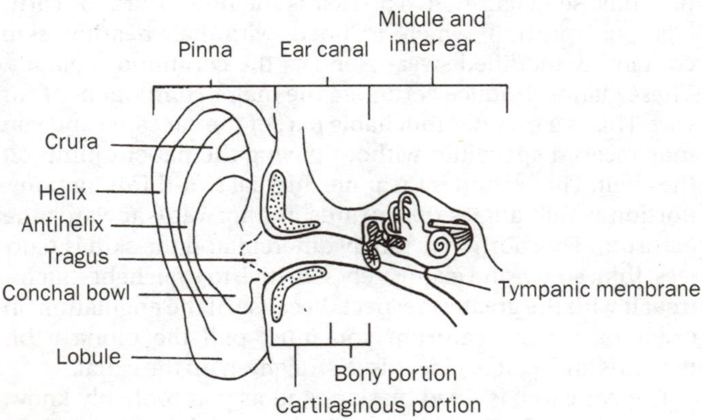

Figure 1.1 The pinna and ear canal

The pinna

Referring to Figure 1.1, see if you can recognize all the different parts of this structure on a colleague. Names to note are the helix, the antihelix with its two superior crura, the tragus, the lobule, and the conchal bowl which leads into the ear canal.

In the embryological stage, the pinna forms from fusion of a collection of little humps, or hillocks, on the side of the head of the developing foetus. A fairly common congenital abnormality is the pre-auricular pit which arises because of incomplete fusion between two of these humps, usually between the helix and the tragus. It can lead into a multiloculated sac which is often a site for infection and abscess formation. Uncommon, grosser abnormalities arise from failure of development or fusion of the humps to form abnormal, small ear remnants, known as microtia.

The ear canal

The ear canal, for clinical purposes, is considered to have two portions; see Figure 1.1. The first is the outer third, or cartilaginous, portion which is lined with hair-bearing skin containing modified sweat glands – the ceruminous glands. These glands produce cerumen, the major component of ear wax. This is a friendly, touchable part of the ear canal and you may insert a speculum without having the patient jump off the chair. The second is the inner, medial two-thirds, or bony, portion which angles downwards and forwards towards the eardrum. This portion is totally different and the skin is hairless, thin, shiny, and exquisitely sensitive to even light touch – treat it with the greatest respect. Because of the angulation, in order to see the eardrum you must pull the pinna a bit upwards and a bit backwards to straighten up the canal.

The ear canal is lined by skin, and as you probably know, skin continually sheds its surface layer of dead skin cells, a process known as desquamation. There has to be a mechanism for clearing all this desquamated debris out of the ear canal. This is achieved by having a pattern of migration from the centre of the drum, outwards to its margins, and then up and out of the ear canal. Any desquamated epithelium, debris, particles, hairs, or wax thus naturally migrate out of the ear canal to be shed into the conchal bowl. Interference with this mechanism, such as cotton bud usage, leads to accumulation and the possibility of having to have the ear canal syringed to get rid of the wax.

The tympanic membrane

Almost all of the tympanic membrane, or eardrum (see Figure 1.2), is made up of a slightly concave, translucent membrane. This larger portion of the membrane is the pars tensa and its margins are well demarcated from the canal walls. It has a smooth, squamous epithelial surface that tends to reflect the light of an otoscope – the light reflex (of no clinical significance). Embedded in the pars tensa is the handle of the malleus (one of the ossicles – see below) and superiorly this has a small, outward-projecting bump – the lateral process. Superiorly to the lateral process there is a small area of the drum which blends into the texture of the bony canal skin without any clear demarcation. This area is the pars flaccida (important to ENT surgeons because sinister ear disease may arise here, for example cholesteatoma; see Chapter 4, page 49).

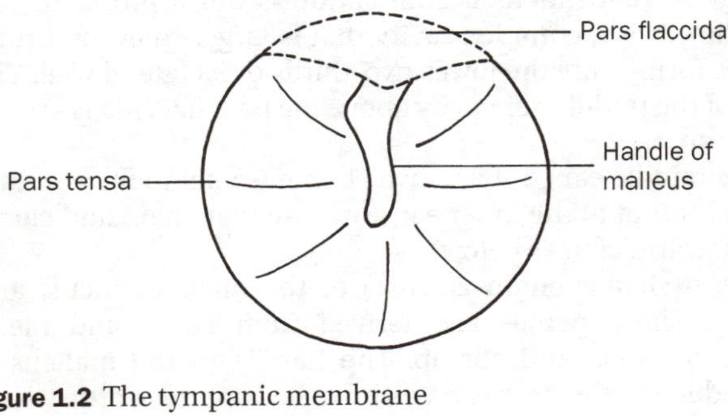

Figure 1.2 The tympanic membrane

Sound waves (energy) are collected and channelled by the pinna into the ear canal. When it is quiet, try cupping your hands around your ears to increase the size of the pinna and notice the increase in amplification of sounds. The canal has a resonating frequency which selectively amplifies sounds of higher frequencies. These collected sound waves set the drum vibrating and, since the handle of the malleus is embedded in the drum, vibrations are transmitted to the ossicular chain of the middle ear.

The middle ear

The complete middle ear cleft (see Figure 1.3) comprises the **eustachian** tube, the middle ear cavity, and the mastoid air cell complex. The middle ear cavity is sometimes called the tympanic cavity – anything beginning tymp- refers to the middle ear, anything beginning myring- refers to the eardrum. The eustachian tube opens into the anterior wall of the middle ear cavity and is only open intermittently to the nasopharynx. On the posterior wall of the middle ear is an opening which leads into the **mastoid air cell complex** within the mastoid portion of the temporal bone. The entire middle ear cleft is lined by respiratory mucosa. For the most part, cilia are absent so that mucus transport towards and down the eustachian tube is relatively inefficient. Fortunately, in the normal middle ear there are only scanty mucus-secreting glands so that mucus accumulation is not a problem. The middle ear is a complex cavity that is larger than the drum, which forms only the lower two-thirds of its lateral wall. The area of the middle ear cavity above the pars flaccida is known as the attic.

The middle ear contains two elements vital to the conduction of sound to the inner ear – an ossicular chain and clean, moist, warm air (see below).

The **ossicular chain** consists of the malleus, incus, and stapes. These names are derived from Latin, and mean hammer, anvil, and stirrup. The handle of the malleus is embedded in the drum and its head lies up in the attic where

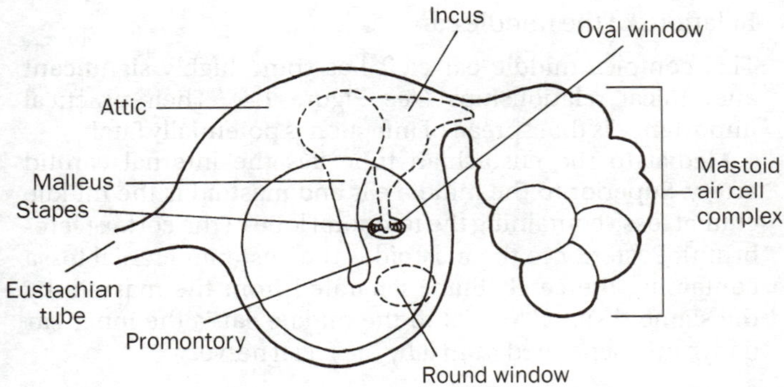

Figure 1.3 The middle ear

it articulates with the incus. The incus has a long process that angles downwards to articulate with the head of the stapes. The stapes enters a recess in the medial wall of the middle ear – the oval window. Here its footplate has a mobile, circumferential joint that closes off the oval window. The inner surface of the footplate is in contact with the fluid of the inner ear. Thus vibrations along the ossicular chain are transmitted into the inner ear for processing.

What goes in must come out, and to accommodate the pressure changes created by vibration of the foot plate there is another mobile window – the round window. This is closed only by fibrous tissue and mucosa and is located on the medial wall of the middle ear just below the oval window. The two windows are separated by a bony bump, the promontory, which houses the basal turn of the coiled cochlea of the inner ear (see below).

Just above the oval window there is another bony hump and this covers the canal in which lies the facial nerve. The facial nerve originates in the brain stem, enters the internal auditory canal, passes over the cochlea, then angles backwards in the middle ear towards the mastoid where it angles inferiorly towards the stylomastoid foramen. Through the foramen it exits from the temporal bone to enter the parotid gland.

Relations of the middle ear

This complex middle ear cleft has some highly significant anatomical relationships (see Figure 1.4). Their practical importance is that spread of infection is potentially fatal.

Medial to the eustachian tube lies the internal carotid artery. Superior to the middle ear and mastoid is the middle cranial fossa containing the temporal lobe of the cortex (cerebrum). Posterior to the mastoid is the posterior cranial fossa containing the cerebellum, separated from the mastoid by the sigmoid sinus. Medial to the middle ear is the inner ear (labyrinth) separated from it by the facial nerve.

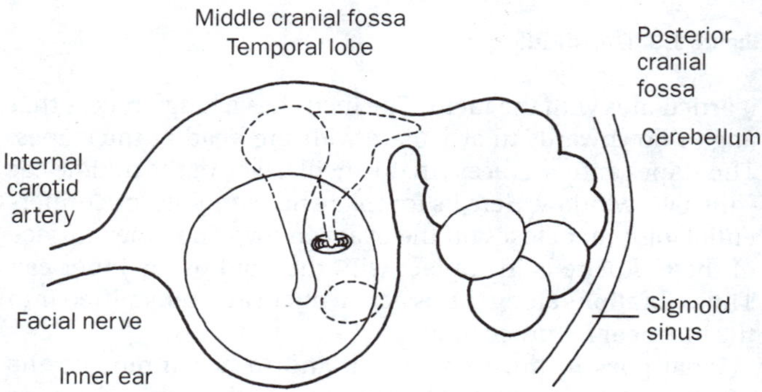

Figure 1.4 Relations of the middle ear

Sound conduction

Why do we need a middle ear when we have an external ear that directs sound wave energy down the ear canal? If you were to stand at the edge of a pool and shout at a friend swimming below the surface,.the message would not be heard since the sound waves bounce off the surface interface, and most of the sound energy is then reflected. In a similar manner, if the sound wave were to impinge directly onto the oval window, most of its energy would be reflected and very little would be transmitted into the inner ear – a situation that is seen clinically when middle ear disease causes ossicular chain discontinuity with a resulting conduction hearing loss of about 50 decibels. To overcome this problem there has to be some mechanism for amplifying the sound wave energy sufficiently to overcome reflection and ensure transmission – this is what the middle ear accomplishes. Sound waves impinge on the tympanic membrane, in which the handle of the malleus is embedded, setting in motion vibrations which are faithfully transmitted along the ossicular chain to the stapes footplate. The tympanic membrane is some seventeen times larger than the stapes footplate, giving an energy amplification of about 17:1. The ossicular chain has an additional lever effect of about 1,3:1. The two together provide a transference enhancement of something like 22:1, sufficient to ensure transmission of the sound wave in its original form into the inner ear where it then travels freely in the cochlear fluids for a distance entirely dependent upon its frequency (this is described later). (See Figure 1.5.)

Two terms that you will need to know in connection with sound wave energy are frequency (pitch), measured in hertz (Hz, cycles per second), and intensity, measured in decibels (dB).

The efficiency of this sound conduction mechanism is dependent on the free vibration of the eardrum and the mobility of the ossicles. It is essential, therefore, that the

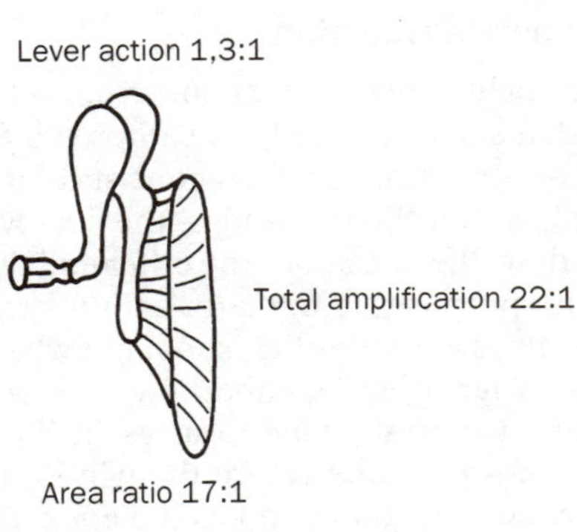

Figure 1.5 Middle ear sound conduction

external and middle ears both contain air. Easy for the outer ear; it is in direct communication with the atmosphere, but the middle ear is a closed system open only to the outside at the whim of the eustachian tube. Air in any closed body cavity is continually absorbed and air in the middle ear is no exception. The eustachian tube is regularly opened by contraction of the palatal muscles, particularly during the act of swallowing, and this allows air to be replaced, consequently equalizing pressure across the tympanic membrane to permit free vibration. Aeration failure from eustachian tube dysfunction not only results in a negative middle ear pressure, but promotes increased production and poor clearance of mucus. The presence of mucus (middle ear effusion) damps down the vibration capability of both the drum and the ossicles.

The inner ear

The inner ear has two functions – hearing and balance. The parts of the ear responsible for these functions – the cochlea for hearing and the semicircular canals, utricle, and saccule for balance – are housed in a labyrinth of fluid-filled tunnels in the dense petrous portion of the temporal bone.

The hearing function

The **cochlea** derives its name from its shape – it looks like a garden snail shell and the Latin word for this is cochlea (see Figure 1.6). Structurally, it consists of a tube doubled over on itself so that the two ends – the oval window and the round window – lie one above the other and the ends are then rolled up for purposes of miniaturization – rather like those irritating things at parties that shoot out when you blow into them. It is easier to understand how the cochlea functions if you think of it straightened out as in Fig. 1.6. The end of the doubled-over tube where the windows are is known as the basal end, the other end as the apex. The fluid in the tube is known as perilymph. Perilymph communicates with cerebrospinal fluid (CSF) through a channel known as the cochlear aqueduct, which is a potential channel for spread of infection into the inner ear from meningitis, which in turn probably explains why deafness is a potential complication of meningitis. The partition between the two tubes is not a membrane but another tube, which contains a different fluid known as endolymph and which has a completely different ionic composition to perilymph. Within this inner endolymphatic compartment is a membrane – the basilar membrane – which supports the hair cells. The hair cells are connected to neurones and the neurones all combine to form the auditory portion of the 8th cranial nerve. (See Figure 1.7.)

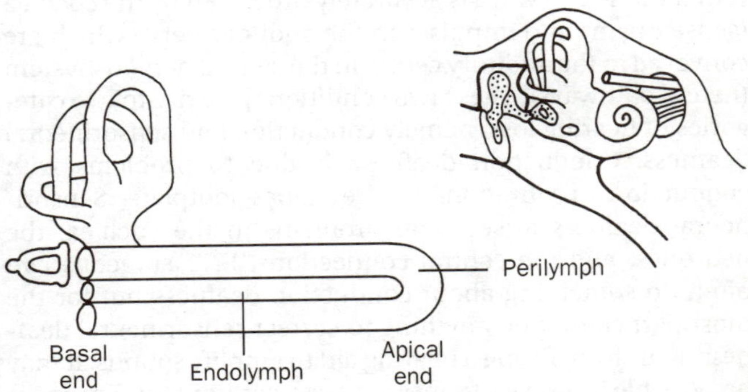

Figure 1.6 The cochlea

The vibrating stapes sends a sound wave through the cochlear fluids, stimulating hair cells which in turn produce a nerve impulse in their neurones. What is special about the cochlea is that each frequency in the sound wave stimulates a different part of the basilar membrane. The basal end responds to high frequencies and the apical end to low frequencies – so-called tonotopic representation. This separation of frequencies is probably what makes it possible for the auditory centre – to which all the nerve impulses eventually travel – to decode the nerve impulses into the sounds that we hear.

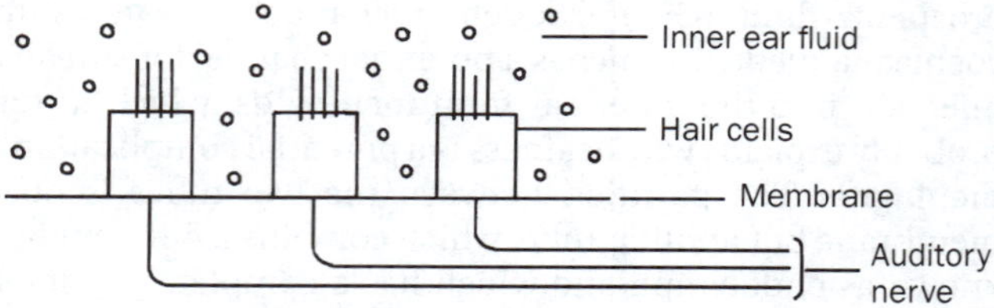

Figure 1.7 Cochlear hair cells

Hearing depends on two conditions being met. The first is that the sound wave is conducted from the outside environment (air) to the inside environment of the cochlea (fluid-filled perilymph and endolymph compartments). The second is that the sound wave is accurately processed by the cochlea (sense organ) into impulses in the auditory nerve which are conveyed to the auditory centre in the central nervous system (neural pathways). These two conditions give rise to two categories of hearing loss, namely conduction and sensorineural deafness. Conduction deafness is due to problems with conduction of vibrations to the stapes footplate. Sensorineural deafness arises from problems in the cochlea, the neurones, and the central connections. ENT surgeons can often do something about conduction deafness but for the most part cannot do anything to correct sensorineural deafness apart from fitting a hearing aid to amplify sounds. It may be possible, however, to insert a cochlear implant. For more information on cochlear implants, see Chapter 2, *Audiology*.

The balance function

The vestibular system (organs of balance) consists of the three semicircular canals, and the utricle and saccule. These organs also have highly specialized hair cells but here the hairs are embedded in a covering 'cap' (cupola); see Figure 1.8. Stimulation of the hair cells to produce a nerve impulse occurs when this cap is displaced by acceleration (utricle), gravity (saccule), or rotation (semicircular canals). These nerve impulses will be interpreted as movement in the vestibular centre in the central nervous system.

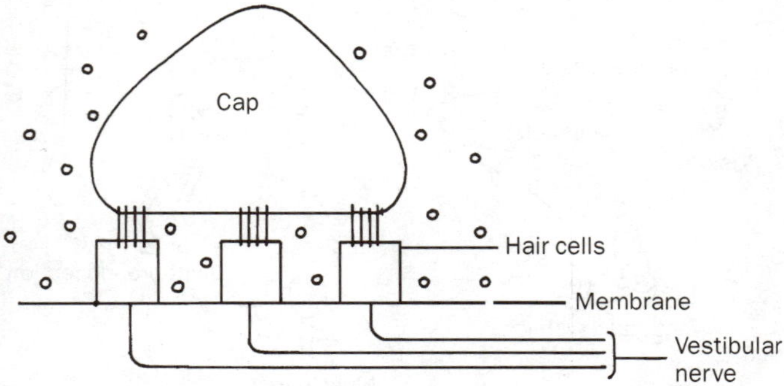

Figure 1.8 Vestibular hair cells

Balance is a constant battle against gravity. It is made more difficult because we stand upright and because we are very mobile – we rotate and we accelerate. There are more central connections for balance than for any of the other senses. Even a mild disturbance in any of these connections gives rise to dizziness – the most incapacitating of all sensory upsets. '**Dizziness**' and '**dizzy spells**' are words patients use in a very non-specific manner. When doctors speak about dizziness they are referring to symptoms such as faintness, blackouts, feelings of imbalance, or falling. They use the word '**vertigo**' for an abnormal sensation of rotation because this is the predominant symptom of vestibular system upsets.

The most important sensory input into the balance system (see Figure 1.9) besides the vestibular system is vision, but muscle tone and joint proprioception from both the neck and the limbs are also significant. This means that symptoms of what we call disequilibrium may not only arise from the organs of balance in the vestibular system of the inner ear, but also from these other sensory inputs.

All this sensory information is co-ordinated by the vestibular nuclei in the brain stem. From here there are connections to both the cerebellum and the cerebrum. The cerebellum co-ordinates the body's responses to changes in sensory input. The cerebrum probably exerts some overall control but is predominantly concerned with our awareness of changes.

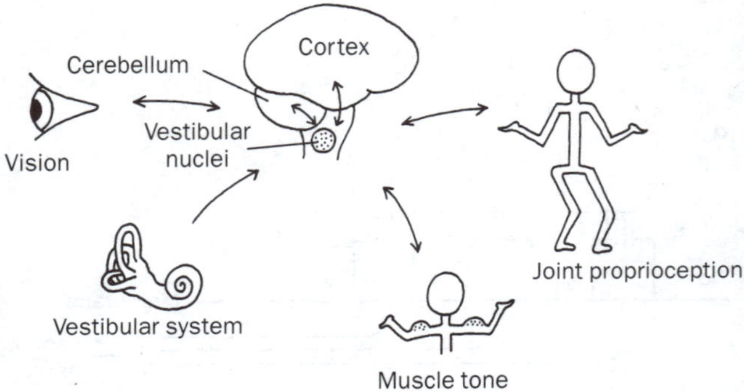

Figure 1.9 The balance system

Rotation

How the vestibular system functions is very complex. For those of you who want to try and understand something about it, the following is a brief description of just one aspect, namely rotation. The first fact to grasp is that within the vestibular system of the inner ear the different receptor organs in each ear are mirror images of each other, each pair having an equal and opposite action. Next consider the resting state. Since gravity is in constant operation (weightlessness induces profound symptoms of seasickness in the uninitiated) there is a constant – and equal on the opposite side – discharge from the receptors even in the resting state – because of gravity they are never 'at rest'. So what happens when movement occurs? Displacement of a receptor in one direction increases this discharge rate and in the other decreases it. The semicircular canals are concerned with rotation movements. When the head rotates, the natural inertia of the fluid in a canal causes the receptor organ to displace in the opposite direction to the head movement and to initiate a change in the discharge rate. Because the semicircular canals in the two ears are mirror images of each other, there will be an increased rate of discharge from one ear and a decreased rate of discharge from the other which is fed into the vestibular nuclei in the brain stem. This is what engineers would call a finely tuned servo-mechanism that enables even small rotation movements to be very accurately monitored. From here this complex input of increased or decreased neurological activity is passed to either other brain-stem motor nuclei or on to higher centres where it is unscrambled, decoded, and translated into some form of instant action response.

One such instant action response regulates eye movements in response to rotation. If the eyes remained in a fixed position in the orbits when the head rotated, the image would be constantly moving across the retina. To overcome this problem, the eyes need to rotate at the same speed but in the opposite direction to the rotation of the head. This is accomplished by what is known as the 'vestibulo-ocular reflex' (VOR), a complex and extensive link in the brain stem between the vestibular and occulomotor nuclei.

When the head rotates there is, however, a comfortable limit as to how far the eye can be swivelled in the opposite direction, and at short, regular intervals a very quick corrective movement returns the eye to the midline for the exercise to commence again. This slow deviation from, and swift return to, the midline is called **nystagmus**. Thus nystagmus is a physiological response to rotation of the head mediated by alterations in the resting discharge rate in the nerves from the receptors in the semicircular canals as rotation movements occur.

A number of pathological processes can alter these resting potentials – infection, trauma, a tumour on the vestibular nerve, ototoxic drugs – and if this happens the brain is fooled into believing that the head is moving, with consequent mobilization of the VOR and nystagmus. Nystagmus is thus one of the clinical signs that indicates the presence of a vestibular disorder. In investigation of vestibular disorders it is often useful to have a recording of the nystagmus. This is obtained using an instrument that detects minute changes in electrical activity as the eyeball moves – an electronystagmograph. The print-out is an electronystagmogram or ENG.

If you are really interested in the vestibular function, you could build up similar pictures of responses to movements of linear or acceleratory nature which are monitored by the otolith organs in the utricle and saccule.

Nerves of hearing and balance

The nerves of hearing (auditory nerve) and balance (vestibular nerve) constitute the 8th cranial nerve, which passes to the brain stem via the internal auditory canal (meatus). This canal is shared with the 7th cranial nerve, the **facial nerve**.

As mentioned earlier, the facial nerve (see Figure 1.10) pursues a winding course intimately related to inner, middle, and outer ear structures. Because ear disease processes may involve the facial nerve to cause facial nerve palsy, investigation and management of facial palsy is usually undertaken by ENT surgeons. There is more about this in Chapter 4, *Core knowledge of ear disorders.* The anatomy of the facial nerve has some clinical relevance because one aspect to the investigation of facial palsy is to try to localize the site of nerve

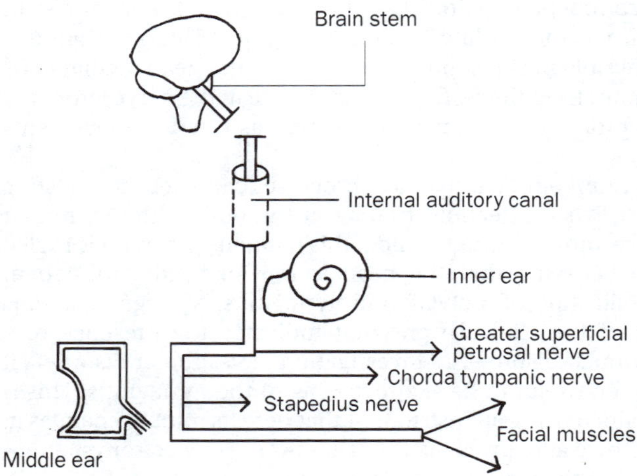

Figure 1.10 Facial nerve anatomy

injury, and testing the function of the various branches of the facial nerve can be useful in doing this:

- The greater superficial petrosal nerve transmits secretomotor fibres to the lacrimal gland.
- The chorda tympani nerve transmits secretomotor fibres to the submandibular gland and returns sensory taste fibres from the anterior two-thirds of the tongue.
- The motor nerve to stapedius muscle is involved in the stapedius reflex (see Chapter 2, *Audiology*).
- The facial nerve terminates in five main branches in the parotid gland that provide motor fibres to all the muscles of the face responsible for facial expression.

2 Audiology

Audiology is an essential complement to otology and encompasses:

- Assessment of hearing disorders
- Assessment of vestibular function
- Assessment of facial nerve palsy
- Prescription and fitting of hearing aids and provision of auditory rehabilitation

Assessment of hearing disorders

With patients who present complaining of hearing loss, or in the case of children suspected of suffering from hearing loss, much can be achieved clinically – history and examination for possible diagnosis, voice testing to gain an idea of the degree of hearing impairment, and use of a tuning fork to differentiate conductive from sensorineural deafness. Once hearing loss is confirmed, patients need to be referred for audiological evaluation to quantify and characterize the hearing loss.

Air-conduction audiogram

On an audiometer one can select pure tones of different frequencies and present these to the patient at different intensities through either headphones or speakers. The patient is asked to identify the air-conduction threshold for each frequency in first one ear and then the other, and these are charted on the audiogram. On the audiogram (see Figure 2.1) the frequencies 250–8 000 cycles per second – Hz – are charted across and the intensities – decibels (dB) – are charted down the chart. Zero hearing loss (0 dB) is biologically defined as the hearing threshold of a normal young adult but decibels also have a physics definition. The intensity of the output of the audiometer can be increased up to 120 dB, above which the sound becomes physically uncomfortable – the hearing discomfort level. (The lay public have difficulty with the concept of a decibel – who doesn't! – and tend to equate it with a percentage, for example 50 dB hearing loss = 50% deaf.)

Bone-conduction audiogram

If a hearing loss is confirmed, the next investigation is a bone-conduction audiogram (cf. tuning fork test). A bone-conduction transducer plugs into the audiometer and this is placed over the mastoid bone. The threshold for each different frequency is determined in a similar manner to the air-conduction threshold and charted on the audiogram. Charting bone-conduction thresholds can be a little confusing, as we all know that normally air conduction is better than bone conduction. The audiometer is calibrated in such a way that 0 dB hearing loss with bone conduction is charted on the same line on the audiogram as 0 dB hearing loss with air conduction. Therefore a patient with a sensorineural hearing loss will have similar air- and bone-conduction thresholds – see Figure 2.1. When the bone-conduction threshold is better than the air-conduction threshold – known as an 'air-bone gap' (see Figure 2.1) – this indicates a conductive hearing loss.

One factor that needs to be taken into consideration with bone conduction is that the sound will be heard equally well in both ears because the sound is conducted through the skull. If one ear has a hearing loss and the other is normal, the apparent bone-conduction threshold in the deafer ear will be better than the true threshold because the sound is being heard in the good ear. To prevent this from happening, the good ear has to be **masked**. Without going into the technicalities of masking, this involves making a louder, but different, sound in the good ear than the intensity of the pure tone being presented to the deaf ear.

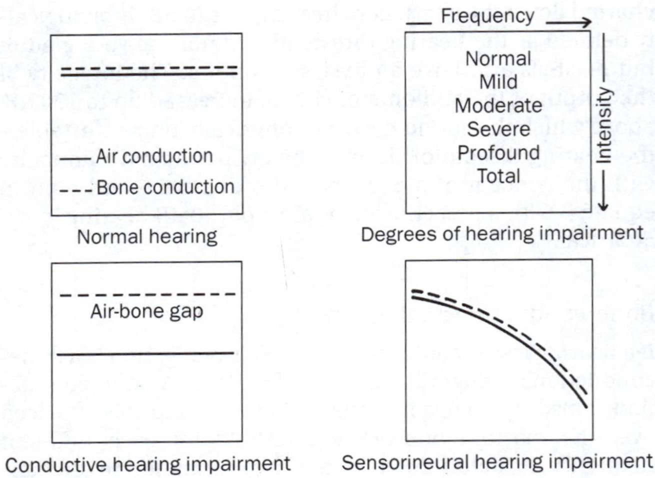

Figure 2.1 Audiometry

Conductive deafness is predominantly an amplification problem. With sensorineural deafness (sensori = hair cells, neural = nerve pathway), there is the added factor that there is nearly always an element of distortion of the sounds heard and this tends to be worse when the neural component is at fault, for example acoustic neuroma.

A **speech audiogram** is the next investigation for sensorineural deafness to try and differentiate between these two components to the deafness. Words can be heard but not understood at the threshold of hearing. It is only when the words are presented through the audiometer at 30 dB above the pure tone threshold that they can be understood. If a list of words is presented at this level to someone with normal hearing, he or she should score 100 per cent correct. Patients with sensorineural deafness due to a hair cell problem will not achieve 100 per cent but should score somewhere close to this, whereas a patient with a nerve pathway problem will achieve nowhere near this score.

Tympanometry

Tympanometry is another routine audiological investigation and as the name implies (tympanum = the middle ear) is an investigation of aspects to middle ear function. A tympanometer can assess three components:

- The mobility of the tympanic membrane which can be hypermobile (atrophy), normal, hypomobile (scarring), or immobile (middle ear effusion or middle ear fibrosis) – see Figure 2.2.
- The middle ear pressure, which can be positive (valsalva), normal, or negative (eustachian tube dysfunction).
- What is called the '**stapedius reflex**'. The stapedius muscle, innervated by a branch of the facial nerve, inserts into the head of the stapes. In response to sound presented through the tympanometer probe at 80 dB or greater above the hearing threshold, there will be a reflex contraction of the muscle (which probably has a protective function for the inner ear) that will show up on a tympanogram as a minute movement of the drum. The presence of a reflex and the threshold at which it is elicited can be determined. If a reflex is absent, the cause is either involvement of the facial

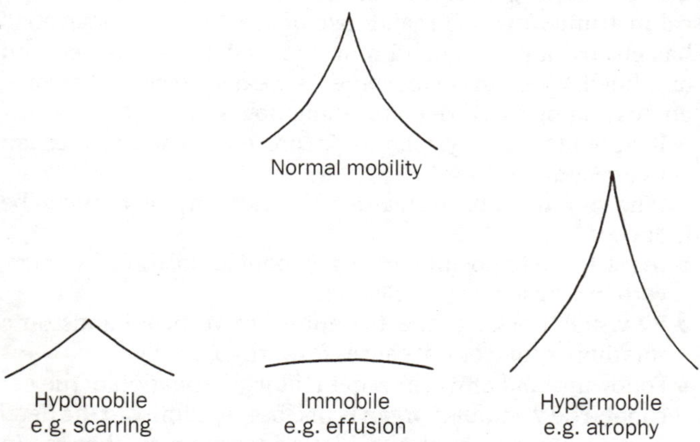

Figure 2.2 Tympanometry

nerve (facial nerve palsy) or an elevation of the hearing threshold (deafness). This is the simplest objective investigation for the hearing threshold.

Brain-stem audiometry

A more complex objective investigation is brain-stem audiometry. This is sometimes needed for the very young or the unco-operative. Using special electrophysiological equipment and electrodes, nerve impulses in the auditory neural pathways that are generated in response to sounds can be detected, amplified, recorded, and analysed to provide information regarding both the hearing threshold and the integrity of the neural pathways – the latter being useful in suspected acoustic neuroma.

Assessment of vestibular function

Nystagmus usually indicates the presence of a disorder of the vestibular component of the balance system (vestibulo-ocular reflex). Nystagmus can be visually observed but more usefully it can be recorded using a special electrophysiological instrument which makes use of the fact that the eyeball has electrical polarity and movements can be detected and amplified. When these movements are displayed and recorded this is known as an electronystagmogram.

If spontaneous nystagmus is present this indicates an active vestibular disorder.

If no spontaneous nystagmus is present, nystagmus can be induced:

- In response to position changes (benign positional vertigo, vertebro-basilar insufficiency).
- By visual 'tracking' of a pendulum or vertical bands on a rotating drum (central causes for vertigo).
- Following cold or warm water (**caloric**) irrigation of the ear canal. The vestibular organ is in close proximity to the deep part of the ear canal and is very sensitive to changes in temperature – see precautions in *Syringing of ears,* Chapter

14, page 189. The caloric test localizes the disorder to one or other ear (vestibular neuronitis, Ménière's disease, trauma).

Although vestibular disorders can usually be diagnosed from the history (see Chapter 5, *A practical approach to ear disorders*), investigation of nystagmus may sometimes provide useful additional information.

Assessment of facial nerve palsy

It is sometimes helpful to try and localize the site of injury in facial nerve palsy. This is done by testing responses of each of the branches of the facial nerve – see *Facial nerve* in Chapter 1, page 16. The stapedius reflex, mentioned above, is the test used for the branch to the stapedius muscle.

It is also useful to know what state the palsied nerve is in – neuropraxia or nerve degeneration – because this relates to the prognosis. Neuropraxia always recovers fully, whereas a significant number of patients who have undergone nerve degeneration never regain full function and are left with problems such as incomplete recovery with facial weakness and re-routing of nerve fibres to give mass movement (synkinesia) or 'crocodile tears'. Sometimes surgical intervention with nerve decompression may be indicated in nerve degeneration to try and improve the prognosis. The state of the nerve is most simply determined by the response to nerve stimulation. The nerve trunk is stimulated and one looks to see whether or not this elicits a muscle twitch. This is done a week after the onset of the palsy because degeneration takes this long to show up on testing. A responsive nerve is in a state of neuropraxia, whereas an unresponsive nerve has undergone degeneration. A more quantitative investigation is electroneuronography which involves recording the impulses generated in the nerve using electrodes and an electrophysiological instrument. This can detect the presence of nerve degeneration much earlier than simple nerve stimulation. It is needed when surgical intervention is contemplated because the earlier this is done the greater the chance of benefit.

Prescription of hearing aids

Bone-conduction hearing aids

Bone-conduction hearing aids are used for conditions in which there is either no external ear canal (congenital microtia with canal atresia, traumatic stenosis) or troublesome recurrent ear infection (active chronic otitis media, mastoid cavities), makes the use of an ordinary hearing aid difficult. Usually a bone-conduction aid uses something similar to the bone-conduction transducer of an audiometer which is held in place with a head band. At their most sophisticated, however, bone-conduction aids are anchored into the skull with titanium screws – bone-anchored hearing aids.

Air-conduction hearing aids

Air-conduction hearing aids originally consisted of a pick-up microphone and amplifier worn on the body which was connected to the output speaker in the ear by a cord. This type of aid is sometimes still used when high amplification is needed or when a patient has problems manipulating very small controls. Modern aids have been miniaturized and are worn either behind the ear or in the ear canal. Both of these have to fit very precisely in the ear canal because any sound leak around the canal 'mould' causes electronic feedback to the pick-up microphone in the aid and a loud whistle or whine. Air-conduction aids vary greatly in sophistication (and hence price!) but can often be tailored to the type of hearing loss. High-tone deafness requires an aid with 'low-tone cut-off' and amplification of high tones – this can also be helped by manipulating the mould to make use of the selective high-tone amplification that occurs in the ear canal. Patients whose hearing is very sensitive to loud sounds can be fitted with aids with automatic 'gain' control.

Hearing aids are simply amplifiers and patients with conductive deafness will benefit most from using them because their problem is simply one requiring a louder sound. When sensorineural deafness is the problem, there is almost always some element of distortion to the sounds heard. Nonetheless, most patients with sensorineural deafness will benefit from using a hearing aid although they may find some hearing situations better than others when using their aid. Audiotherapy involves working with patients so that they derive the maximum benefit from their aid. There will be the occasional patient who finds amplified distortion intolerable. These patients may require to be taught additional skills, such as lip reading, to help them overcome their deafness handicap and to use their aid at lesser amplification.

Cochlear implants

Cochlear implants are used when there has been near total loss of hair cells but the neural pathways are still intact. These very sophisticated (and hence very expensive!) devices consist of a pick-up component that converts sound into electrical impulses and directs these to a multichanneled electrode (high tones to one end, low tones to the other) which is implanted into the cochlea. The electrodes directly stimulate the nerve fibres and the generated impulses are interpreted as sound in the auditory centre. If one considers that 30 000 hair cells are being replaced by 22 electrodes, the quality of the sound can be deduced but with intensive training the quality of an otherwise totally deaf patient's life can be dramatically improved. Many patients are able to understand speech by using a combination of the sound heard and visual clues (lip reading).

3 Structured approach to examination of the ear

The summary in Table 3.1 is the basis for learning how to examine an ear, something that is not usually well taught and which is a difficult skill to master. The rest of this chapter expands on the summary providing both practical details and explaining the significance of findings.

Table 3.1 Aids to examination in otology

The external ear
Normality is determined by exclusion of abnormality. There are really only three categories of abnormality:

- Deformities
  - congenital: remember possibility of deafness
  - old acquired: e.g. cauliflower ear
  - recent acquired, traumatic: e.g. haematoma
    inflammatory: e.g. perichondritis
    neoplastic: e.g. squamous cell or basal cell carcinoma
- Inflammatory swelling
  - mastoiditis: abnormal middle ear
  - lymphadenitis: normal middle ear
- Surgical scars: tympanoplasty, mastoidectomy

The ear canal
Normality is determined by exclusion of abnormality. There are really only four categories of abnormality:

- Wax – diagnosis: **wax**

Table 3.1 continued

- Foreign body – diagnosis: **foreign body**
- Infection – diagnosis: **otitis externa** – localized (furuncle), generalized
- Others
  - uncommon conditions, e.g. exostoses, hyperkeratosis, stenosis, atresia
  - a defect in the posterior wall opening into a mastoid cavity

The eardrum

Normality is determined by exclusion of abnormality. There are really only five categories of abnormality:

- Inflammation – diagnosis: **acute otitis media**
- Perforation:
  - infected – diagnosis: **active chronic otitis media**
  - dry – diagnosis: **inactive chronic otitis media**
- Scarred – diagnosis: **healed otitis media**
- Retracted – diagnosis: **otitis media with effusion**
- Others:
  - uncommon conditions, e.g. uninfected cholesteatoma

The hearing

Normal hearing is determined by an accurate response to your **whispered voice test**.

If the response is inaccurate, proceed to test with your **normal voice** – moderate hearing impairment – or your **loud voice** – severe hearing impairment.

Use a **tuning fork** to determine whether the hearing impairment is **conductive** or **sensorineural**.

Step 1

Begin with a general examination of the head from the front, focus in on the ears. Are both ears in a normal position?

Low-set and anteriorly displaced ears are representative of some of the congenital abnormalities that fall under the general term ‘funny-looking kid’, or FLK. These children are best referred to a paediatrician or geneticist for definition of the abnormality, as there may be other more significant features to the abnormality.

Step 2

View from the side, focus in on the ear. Are both ears normal? If not, is it possible to define the abnormalities when each ear is examined in turn?

Congenital deformity. The significance of finding a congenitally abnormal ear is that these are usually associated with deafness – either conductive or sensorineural. If only one ear is affected, it is essential to have the hearing in the other ear assessed as soon as practical. If both ears are affected, referral to an ENT specialist is mandatory, as hearing aids will need to be fitted before one year of age if there is any hearing impairment. Good hearing is essential for normal speech development. Children develop speech as they mimic the sounds that they hear and if they cannot hear well, their speech development will be retarded or even absent. They develop vocabulary and understanding of words through use of speech and hearing. Since humans think in words, a restricted or absent vocabulary will impair intellectual development.

A more common abnormality is the pre-auricular sinus, usually situated just above the tragal cartilage. These sinuses have the potential to become infected and form an abscess.

Old acquired deformity. Not much can be done for these patients but the significance lies in possible stenosis of the ear canal. If obstructed, the accumulation of desquamated epithelium in the canal may eventually lead to an expanding, destructive mass trapped in the ear canal.

Recent acquired deformity – traumatic. Lacerations are obvious and may require suture. Of more significance is a haematoma of the pinna. If this is not adequately drained, it may potentially heal with fibrosis and contracture to produce the deformity known as a 'cauliflower ear'.

Recent acquired deformity – inflammatory. A painful, swollen, inflamed pinna is caused by underlying perichondritis. If this condition is not promptly and adequately treated, it has the same potential for subsequent deformity.

Recent acquired deformity – neoplastic. The pinna is one of the common sites in the head and neck for development of basal cell and squamous cell carcinoma. Any non-healing ulcers should be regarded suspiciously.

Inflammatory swelling. Inflammatory swelling behind the ear can be caused by either mastoiditis or lymphadenitis. Mastoiditis is always accompanied by some abnormality of the middle ear – middle ear effusion, frank otitis media, or active chronic otitis media. In the absence of any abnormality, it is probably a lymphadenitis and a primary source of infection, usually in the scalp, should be sought.

Surgical scars. These scars may be either behind the ear or in front above the tragal cartilage, and indicate that either a tympanoplasty (middle ear and eardrum reconstruction) or a mastoidectomy have been performed. They provide a clue as to what to expect when examining the ear canal or the eardrum. A successful tympanoplasty will usually leave the drum scarred, whereas if unsuccessful, there will still be a perforation. There may be no signs to see after a simple mastoidectomy but a radical mastoidectomy, performed for cholesteatoma, will have opened the mastoid cavity into the ear canal by removing the posterior wall of the canal. It is surprisingly easy to overlook a mastoid cavity, probably because the instinct when using an otoscope is to look deep and anteriorly for the eardrum. Knowing that there has been mastoid surgery before looking with the otoscope makes it less likely that a mastoid cavity will be missed.

Step 3

Now take the otoscope! Before you start using it, you need to check that it works by switching it on and checking that the bulb delivers a good light – you will have great difficulty distinguishing any of the subtle features that you need to see unless the light is bright. Select the largest size speculum that will fit into the ear canal. The field of view through an otoscope is very narrow and to build up a composite picture you have to move the speculum around and piece together all of the separate images. The larger the speculum, the less it has to be moved around.

To see into the ear canal it has to be straightened. This is done by taking hold of the pinna and gently pulling it outwards and backwards with a little up or down displacement as needed. If this causes discomfort, it is an indication of possible otitis externa. Before inserting the speculum into the ear canal, inspect the opening to the canal. A furuncle may arise in the hair-bearing area here – classified as **localized otitis externa**. Furuncles are easy to miss unless looked for, and squashing them with a speculum is very painful. Inspecting the entrance to the canal will also reveal any discharge that will need to be mopped or syringed before anything meaningful can be seen.

While still holding the pinna, gently insert the speculum into the canal, all the time looking through the otoscope to see where you are going. Do hairs obstruct your view? Gently manoeuvre the speculum past them. Does wax obscure your view? Can you see adequately past it or are you going to have to remove it?

Step 4

Once you can see the ear canal clearly the question you have to answer is 'Is the ear canal normal?'. This is determined by excluding any abnormality.

Wax and foreign bodies should be obvious and are best removed by syringing.

If the canal walls are inflamed, desquamating, and swollen or if there is an accumulation of wet debris in the canal, the diagnosis is **generalized otitis externa**.

There are a few **uncommon conditions** that occur in the ear canal. One of these occurs in people who swim a lot in cold water, who develop 'swimmer's exostoses' – nodular, bony protrusions from the deep bony portion of the canal. Another is hyperkeratosis – an accumulation of desquamated squamous epithelium in the deep ear canal resulting from failure of the normal migratory process that 'self-cleanses' the canal. Stenosis of the canal can be either congenital or acquired but atresia is always congenital. If a radical mastoidectomy has been performed, the posterior wall of the ear canal will have been removed, and you should be able to see backwards and upwards into an open mastoid cavity. These open cavities can be the source of problems by either filling up with wax or becoming chronically infected.

Step 5

Having established the status of the ear canal, the next step is to examine the eardrum. To do this you need to angle the otoscope speculum a little forwards until you can see the drum. The eardrum is the window to the middle ear and all of the middle ear disorders can be diagnosed by the characteristic appearances that they impart to the drum. A normal eardrum indicates a normal middle ear, although it will not provide information about the essential hearing function of the ear, which has to be assessed after otoscopy has been carried out.

There are two questions that you have to answer at this point. The first question is 'Is the drum intact?'. Examine the drum closely and move your speculum tip around until you have been able to see all of it. The second question is 'Is the drum normal?'. To answer this, you need to think about what you are seeing.

A normal eardrum (see Figure 3.1) is usually described as having a smooth reflective surface with the contour a little indrawn and incorporating the handle of the malleus in the upper part of the pars tensa. The handle of the malleus is

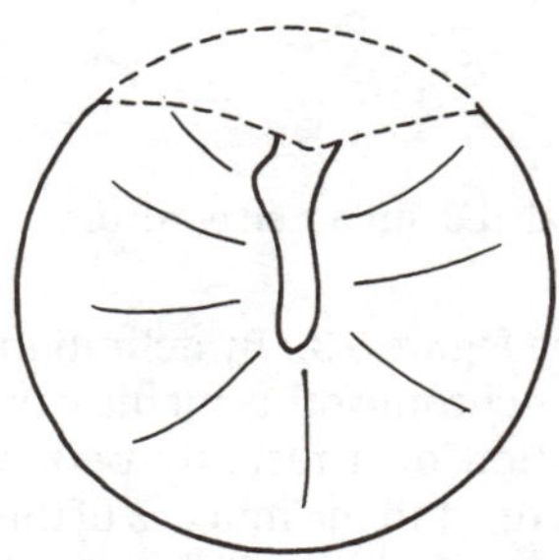

Figure 3.1 Intact normal eardrum

recognized by looking for the small lateral projection at its upper end that marks the division between pars tensa and pars flaccida (which is often very insignificant).

However, there are so many variations to the appearance of a normal eardrum that this latter question is best answered by excluding abnormality. There are really only five categories of abnormality, each representing one of the middle ear disease processes. It helps to be dogmatic about these appearances because once again there are so many variations to each of the abnormalities.

Inflammation. As a general rule inflammation of the drum (see Figure 3.2) is indicative of **otitis media**. The inflammation of otitis media starts with hypervascularity, goes through a stage of generalized inflammation to the late stage of the inflamed, 'bulging' drum. This is not, unfortunately, infallible and sometimes you will be caught out by inflammation of the drum from variations of otitis externa. Pneumatic otoscopy, which will be mentioned later, helps to distinguish the two, as the drum will be what we call 'mobile' if the cause is otitis externa.

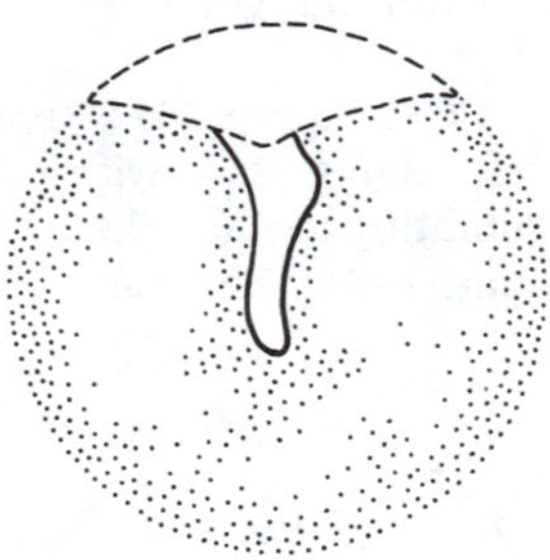

Figure 3.2 Abnormal: red, inflamed eardrum

Perforation. (See Figure 3.3.) By definition, a perforation in the drum indicates chronic otitis media – unless it is a recent traumatic perforation or a recently perforated acute otitis media! If the ear is dry and the mucosa of the middle ear, seen through the perforation, is not inflamed, this is an **inactive chronic otitis media**. If the ear is discharging and the middle ear mucosa is inflamed – there may even be visible granulation tissue on the perforation margins – then this is an **active chronic otitis media**. It is helpful for descriptive purposes to try to define the size of the perforation – 20 per cent, 50 per cent, and so on.

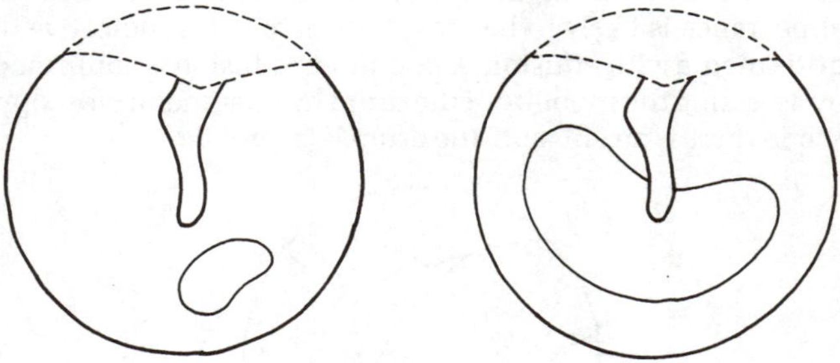

Figure 3.3 Abnormal: perforations

Scarred. (See Figure 3.4.) An intact but scarred eardrum is indicative of **healed otitis media**. These scars may be visible fibrosis or may have become calcified, when they have an appearance described as 'chalk patches'. An atrophic scar in which there is loss of the middle layer of the drum gives rise to the appearance of a transparent patch in the drum described as a healed perforation.

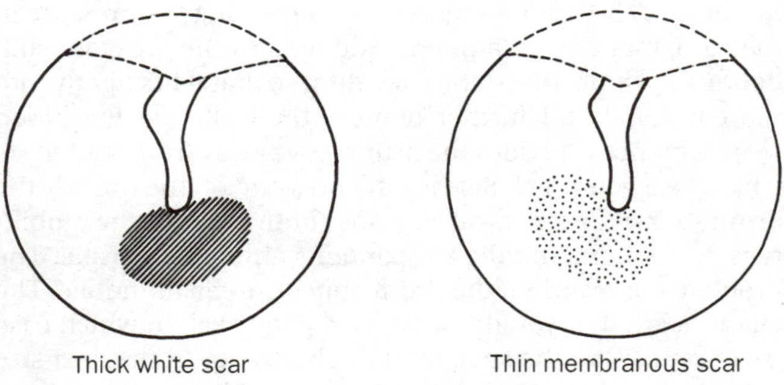

Figure 3.4 Abnormal: scarred

Retracted. (See Figure 3.5.) Retraction of the drum results from a negative middle ear pressure, after obstruction of the eustachian tube, which sucks the drum inwards. It is recognized by looking both at the angulation of the handle of the malleus – which becomes more horizontal than vertical – and anteriorly at the margin of the drum where the 'sucked-in' appearance is likely to be most noticeable. It is indicative of **otitis media with effusion**. A middle ear effusion is confirmed by assessing the mobility of the drum by pneumatic otoscopy. When there is an effusion, the drum is immobile.

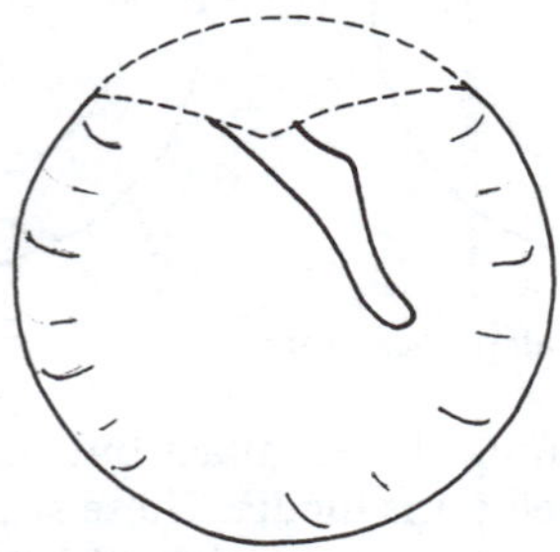

Figure 3.5 Abnormal: retracted eardrum

Pneumatic otoscopy. This is a useful technique to master as it provides the essential additional information sometimes needed to confirm a diagnosis and basically assesses the mobility of the drum in response to changing the pressure in the ear canal. Attach a pneumatic bulb to the otoscope and depress it a little. Insert the speculum so that it fits tightly into the ear canal and further depress the bulb. Do the blood vessels blanch and does the drum move away from you? If so, you have a good seal. Release the pressure on the bulb. Is the drum sucked towards you? If it does both of these, the mobility is normal, the middle ear contains air and is normal. The problem comes when the drum appears to be immobile. The chances are that you do not have a good seal, in which case try to reposition the speculum or change up to the next size speculum and try again. If the drum is still immobile and you are sure that you have a good seal, either there is a **perfora-**

tion which you have missed (easy to do – which is why it is important to perform this manoeuvre) or there is a middle ear effusion – **otitis media with effusion** (these sometimes have a relatively normal-looking drum and are also easily missed).

Others. (See Figure 3.6.) Is there something else about the appearance of the deep ear canal or drum that makes you wonder whether there is another disease process present? A granulation tissue polyp in the deep ear canal over the eardrum, or even filling the ear canal, often hides an underlying infected cholesteatoma. Cholesteatoma usually presents only once it is infected as an active chronic otitis media, when it is difficult to diagnose unless squamous epithelium can be seen in the middle ear through the perforation. Occasionally it will present as deafness without infection, when it may be possible to identify from the presence of a collection of whitish, hyperkeratotic debris in what looks like a pit or a perforation. Recent trauma or acute pressure changes may cause bleeding in the middle ear, imparting a bluish/black appearance to the drum, an appearance known as a haemotympanum.

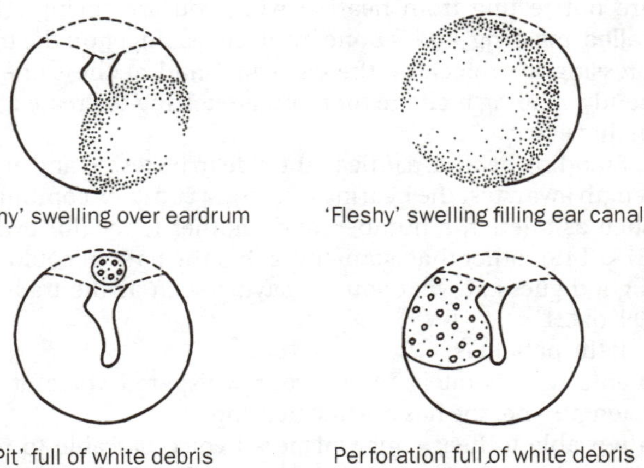

Figure 3.6 Abnormal: others

Step 6

Hearing. Examination of the ear is not complete until the hearing has been assessed. In the clinical setting the hearing threshold should be considered as being in the range of:

- normal hearing
- moderate hearing loss (hearing impairment)
- severe deafness (deaf)

Perhaps the most useful and easy to administer test to determine the hearing threshold is one based on the fact that if you have normal hearing you should be able to make out what is said to you in a whisper from halfway across the room. If you have a hearing impairment, the person speaking has to come a bit closer and speak in a more normal voice. If you are deaf, the person has to come close and speak very loudly for you to make out what has been said.

Step 7

Stand behind the patient and test the hearing in each ear by a 'Repeat after me' voice test. Since you need to test the hearing in each ear separately, you have to prevent the ear that you are not testing from hearing what you are saying. This is called 'masking' and is done by placing a finger on the tragus, pressing it to occlude the ear canal and at the same time gently rubbing it all the time you are testing to create a noise in that ear.

Standing behind, a little to the side to be tested and at arm's length away, test the hearing by using a complex combination such as a letter, a number, and another letter (for example B7K, T4S) rather than something that the patient could make a good guess at what you are saying such as the traditional '99' or '21'.

If the patient is:

- able to accurately repeat your whispered voice at arm's length – he/she has **normal hearing**.
- not able to hear your whispered voice but able to repeat your normal voice at arm's length – he/she has a **hearing impairment** (moderate hearing loss).

- not able to hear your normal voice but able to repeat your loud voice at arm's length – he/she is **deaf** (severe hearing loss).

It will be found that children are reluctant to co-operate with a 'Repeat after me' test. This can be overcome by asking them to do something such as touching their nose, or pointing to their mouth in the same sequence of whispered voice, normal voice, loud voice. You may find that you cannot mask younger children while you are testing them, but at least you will be able to get an impression as to where their hearing threshold lies.

Step 8

If there is any hearing impairment, testing with a tuning fork may indicate whether the deafness is conductive or sensorineural. The tuning fork (Rinne) test is useful, but unfortunately not always reliable and is not usually possible when dealing with children. The importance of carrying out a tuning fork test is that although conductive deafness is usually associated with a visible disease process, this is not always so (for example otosclerosis) and for conductive deafnesses there is the possibility of surgical correction, whereas a sensorineural deafness probably indicates the need for a hearing aid. Points to note are:

- Air conduction better than bone conduction – the tone heard when the tuning fork is held next to the pinna sounds louder than when the base of the tuning fork is pressed against the mastoid bone. This indicates that the conductive mechanism is intact.
- Bone conduction better than air conduction – the tone heard when the tuning fork is held next to the pinna sounds softer than when the base of the tuning fork is pressed against the mastoid bone. This indicates an impairment in the conductive mechanism.

Step 9

Assessment of hearing in babies is a highly skilled procedure that is usually performed by specially trained audiologists. The medical practitioner can obtain a fairly good idea as to whether or not there is a hearing problem by asking the parent or caregiver questions relating to both hearing ability and speech development appropriate for age. The questions to ask for the different ages are given in Table 3.2.

Table 3.2 Questions for use in assessing hearing in babies

Baby only a few weeks old:
Does your baby appear to be listening to you when you talk or sing?
Does your baby open his or her eyes or blink when there is a noise?

Baby about six months old:
Does your baby enjoy your talking or playing word games with him or her?
Does your baby try to see where a noise is coming from by turning his or her eyes or head towards the sound?

Baby about nine months old:
Does your baby appear to enjoy babbling and making other noises?
Does your baby appear to respond to even very soft sounds?

Baby about a year old:
Is your baby beginning to say baby words?
Does your baby respond when you say his or her name and the names of things he or she plays with?

Baby about a year and a half old:
Is your baby beginning to use simple words?
Does your baby pick up or point to things around the house when you ask him or her to do this?

Babies of two years or more:
Is your baby putting words together and trying to talk to you?
Do you think your baby can hear normally even when you speak to him or her in a very soft voice?

Step 10

Piecing together all the information obtained from the history regarding the ear complaint, the findings on examination, and the presence of any hearing loss should enable a diagnosis to be made and a treatment or management plan to be formulated.

4 Core knowledge of ear disorders

The external ear

Impacted wax

Ear wax consists of sebaceous and ceruminous gland secretions combined with hairs and desquamated skin – ear canal epithelium migrates outwards from the drum and deep parts of the canal. The wax varies in colour and consistency and it is normal to have some wax in the outer part of the ear canal. Wax probably has some bactericidal action and may provide some protection for the ear canal. Attempts to 'clean' the ear often simply push any accumulated wax deeper into the canal. Impaction of wax also tends to occur in very dry climates.

Remember that wax dissolves in water. Therefore if wax needs to be removed it is best done by syringing – see Chapter 14, page 189. Indications for removal of wax are a need to see the drum, discomfort in the ear canal, or deafness from impaction.

Otitis externa

Otitis externa is described as being localized (a furuncle) or generalized and may occasionally develop complications (cellulitis, adenitis, perichondritis, necrotizing otitis externa). It may be caused by infection (bacterial, fungal, viral) or by allergy (dermatitis). The pathological process is either inflammation and abscess formation in a hair follicle (furuncle – common) or inflammation of the skin and subcutaneous tissues of the canal causing oedema/induration and increased epithelial desquamation (common). Infection may spread into surrounding soft tissue (cellulitis) and there may be adjacent lymphadenitis – pre-auricular, postauricular, subauricular – or it may spread to involve the perichondrium of the auricular cartilages (perichondritis – uncommon). In a diabetic or immunocompromised patient, pseudomonal infection may spread rapidly into the surrounding temporal bone and beyond (necrotizing otitis externa – uncommon). The symptoms and signs relate to the pathological process, its site, and the extent.

Symptoms
- Itching/irritation
- Pain
- 'Blocked ear'
- Discharge

Signs
- Tenderness on manipulating the pinna or tragus
- Inflammation and swelling – localized or generalized
- Desquamation and accumulation of debris
- Purulent discharge
- Conduction deafness
- Cellulitis
- Tender lymph nodes
- Swollen, inflamed, tender pinna (perichondritis)
- Ulceration, granulation tissue (necrotizing otitis externa)

Treatment
- Cleaning – syringing (see Chapter 14)
- Installation of:
  - something soothing: glycerine/ichthammol either as drops or soaked into a cotton wool wick gently inserted into the ear canal
  - something antiseptic: tinct. Merthiolate® ear drops
  - something anti-inflammatory: steroid-containing ear

drops (these are usually combined with an antibiotic)
– something specific: antifungal drops or creams

- Cellulitis requires antibiotics. Perichondritis requires IV antibiotics. Necrotizing otitis externa requires high-dose specific IV antibiotics and debridement surgery.

Foreign bodies

Small children tend to put things into their own and other children's ears. Sometimes the tips fall off cotton buds, and sometimes insects crawl into ears. It is best to attempt to remove all of these by syringing rather than by trying to hook them out as the latter method usually hurts the child and makes subsequent attempts almost impossible. If unsuccessful, refer to an ENT service or, if unavailable, attempt removal under anaesthetic.

Deformities of the pinna and/or canal

Congenital

- Minor:
  - Cosmetic deformities such as prominent (bat) ears
  - Pre-auricular sinuses (pits). Debris may accumulate and become infected to form an abscess requiring drainage. These sinus tracts need to be excised once the infection has resolved.
- Major:
  - Degrees of what is called microtia with severe deformity of the pinna and stenosis or atresia of the canal. The importance of these major deformities lies in the resulting conductive hearing loss. If this is bilateral, there is an urgency to refer the infant to a specialist service so that management of the deafness can be begun early enough to permit speech development.

Acquired

- Lacerations, burns, etc. produce defects and scarring

(cosmetic).

- Haematomas beneath the perichondrium cause cartilage necrosis (cosmetic, 'cauliflower ear'). Haematomas should be aspirated or a suction drainage tube inserted. If unable to aspirate the haematoma, refer urgently to a specialist service (Plastics, ENT).
- Trauma involving the canal causes fibrosis with subsequent stenosis which interferes with the normal epithelial migration out of the canal. Debris accumulates and can act as a focus for infection. Stenosis requires referral for remedial surgery.

Neoplastic

- The prominent, exposed pinna is a common site for development of basal cell and squamous cell carcinoma. Remember this in consideration of any persistent ulceration.

The middle ear

An overall concept of middle ear disorders may be gained from consideration of the diagram in Table 4.1 below.

Table 4.1 Middle ear disease

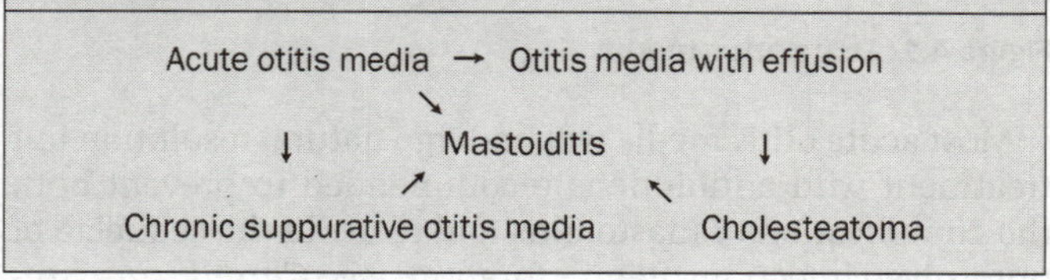

Acute otitis media

Acute otitis media most commonly occurs in young children – peak incidence one to two years – but it can occur at any age. Although often precipitated by a cold or other viral upper respiratory tract infection, it is usually a secondary bacterial infection (**Haemophilus influenzae**, **Streptococcus pneumoniae**, **Streptococcus pyogenes**) that involves the mucous membrane of the middle ear cleft. The infected mucosa produces a mucopurulent exudate which initially drains away down the eustachian tube. When inflammatory swelling obstructs the eustachian tube, a middle ear empyema develops, the inflamed tympanic membrane 'bulges' and may perforate. (See Figure 4.1.) Complications occur when infection becomes trapped within the mastoid air cells – see *Mastoiditis*, page 51.

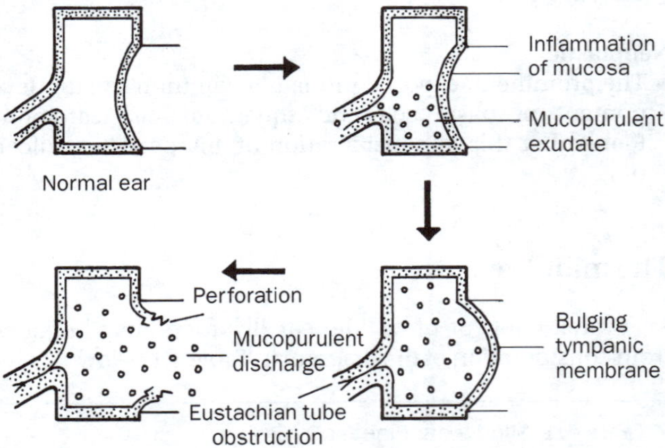

Figure 4.1 Acute otitis media

Most acute otitis media will undergo natural resolution but treatment with antibiotic is recommended to prevent both the complication of mastoiditis and to avoid the sequelae of unresolved infection after perforation – see *Chronic suppurative otitis media*, page 46.

Otitis media with effusion

The eustachian tube has two functions – aeration of the middle ear cleft and drainage of any middle ear secretion.

Middle ear effusions develop when tube function is impaired and this most commonly occurs in children following an episode of otitis media. In many children it takes some time before the middle ear regains normal aeration. Ventilation failure arises either because the middle ear mucosa continues to produce an excess of mucus which 'floods' the eustachian tube and prevents ascent of air, or because the mucosal lining of the tube remains oedematous to cause a mechanical blockage. If the middle ear cannot be ventilated, any residual air is absorbed to create what is called a 'negative middle ear pressure' and mucus accumulates. This impairs vibration of both the drum and the ossicular chain, causing a conductive deafness (which needs to be assessed). The presence of mucus imparts a 'dull', somewhat pinkish appearance to the drum which is generally retracted and immobile. See Figure 4.2.

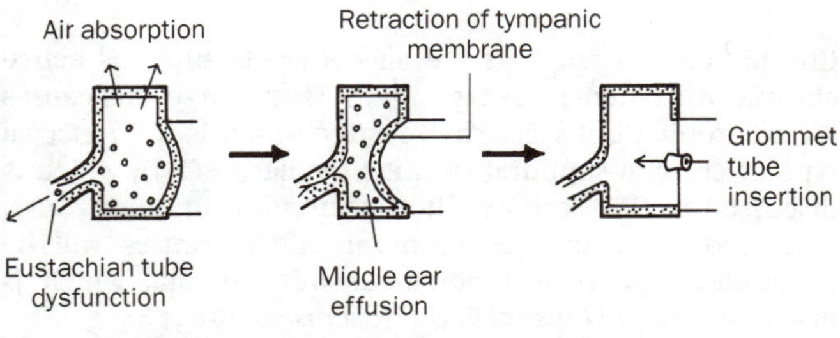

Figure 4.2 Otitis media with effusion

In children, natural resolution is usual given time but there are two problems with expectant management:

- The first is the effect of a persistent hearing impairment on the child's speech and intellectual development. This is managed by inserting a minute ventilation tube through the drum (often known as a grommet tube because of its shape) to aerate the middle ear and hence restore hearing. These tubes usually extrude spontaneously after a few months.
- The second is the effect of a persistent negative middle ear pressure on the retracted drum. The overstretched drum

may become atrophic or a retraction pocket may form – see *Cholesteatoma,* page 49.

In adults, middle ear effusions are uncommon, sometimes encountered after episodes of otitis media and occasionally seen after barotrauma (flying, diving). In adults the effusion is usually serous rather than mucoid (because there are fewer mucus-secreting glands in the adult middle ear mucosa) and this imparts a yellowish colour to the drum.

> In adults with middle ear effusion suspicion has to be high of mechanical obstruction of the eustachian tube by a tumour in the nasopharynx.

Chronic suppurative otitis media

Chronic discharging ears are all better classified as **active chronic otitis media** (see Figure 4.3). There are several causes for a chronic discharge. The most common is the mucosal type of chronic suppurative otitis media (CSOM), which is discussed in this section. Cholesteatoma is another cause, discussed next, and, uncommonly, other causes will be encountered such as tuberculous otitis media, which is discussed under *Unusual middle ear disease,* page 53.

Not all cases of acute otitis media that have progressed as far as perforation resolve. There are two reasons for this:

First, while the body defence mechanisms are clearing the middle ear of the bacteria that caused the acute infection, it becomes colonized by coliform bacteria (Proteus, Klebsiella, *Escherchia coli,* Pseudomonas), which find their way in through the perforation. The body appears to be fairly tolerant of these gut commensals and once they establish in the middle ear, infection persists for a long time with continuous production of mucopurulent discharge (otorrhoea).

Second, changes may occur at the perforation margin which will prevent closure of the perforation during the healing phase. Ideally, the raw margins of the perforation –

remember that there is a mucosal surface on the inside of the drum and a squamous surface on the outside – should regenerate and grow across the defect to close it. This doesn't always happen and sometimes the squamous epithelium on the outside of the drum forms a junction with the mucosa on the inside to create a 'sealed' margin to the perforation. The perforation has now healed but it has healed 'open' rather than closed. Once this has occurred, the perforation will remain open even after infection is controlled to create a state then known as **inactive chronic otitis media**. This is the origin of the definition that any ear with a perforation is classified as **chronic otitis media**.

A further aspect to chronic middle ear infection is that a persistent perforation contributes to conductive deafness. The degree of conductive deafness will be even greater if there is either osteitis and erosion of individual ossicles during the stage of infection, or fixation of the ossicular chain by fibrosis during the healing phase.

Treatment involves a combination of aural toilet and instillation of ear drops, supplemented by use of antibiotics.

Aural toilet and instillation of ear drops are used in an attempt to render the middle ear environment hostile to

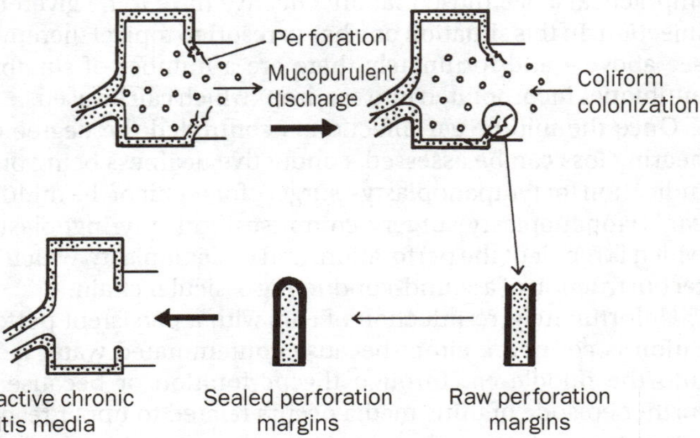

Figure 4.3 Active chronic otitis media

infecting organisms. This is achieved by drying (see *Dry mopping of ears,* Chapter 14) and instilling either acidification agents (acetic acid drops) or antiseptic drops (boracic ear drops) – see *Instilling ear drops,* Chapter 14. Sometimes these inexpensive preparations are not effective and a specific antibiotic has to be used in an ear drop. The more frequently the ear is cleaned and ear drops are instilled, the more effective treatment is likely to be.

It is sometimes difficult to get the ear clean by dry mopping alone and sometimes patients are not co-operative enough to do it adequately. In these circumstances syringing is a very effective way of cleaning out all the infected debris and mucopurulent secretions – see *Syringing of ears,* Chapter 14.

If it appears likely that dry mopping and ear drops will be ineffective, then systemic antibiotics have to be given. This situation applies to most children and also when there is only a very small perforation. The antibiotic selected will have to be one that is effective against a mixed coliform infection. Some of these organisms are sensitive to easily given broad-spectrum antibiotics (Augmentin® – if available – amoxycillin, or co-trimoxazole), but many are resistant. When resistant organisms predominate, systemic administration of the specific antibiotic required (gentamicin or cephalosporins) is usually impractical since those that are effective have to be given by injection. In this situation one has to resort to topical therapy – see above – and fortunately there are a number of suitable antibiotics incorporated into ear drops which can be used.

Once the middle ear infection is controlled the degree of hearing loss can be assessed, conductive deafness being one indication for tympanoplasty – surgery for repair of the middle ear. Tympanoplasty surgery comprises both myringoplasty, which is repair of the perforation, and ossiculoplasty, which is reconstruction of a sound-conducting ossicular chain.

Unfortunately, re-infection of ears with a persistent perforation is common, either because contaminated water gets into the middle ear through the perforation or because a further episode of otitis media occurs related to upper respiratory tract infection. Another indication for tympanoplasty would be to close the perforation to prevent re-infection.

Once the acute infection of otitis media has settled, chronic mucosal middle ear infection is painless. The onset of pain in a chronic discharging ear is an indication that there has been spread of infection from mucosa into underlying bone, particularly in the mastoid, and mastoiditis – see below – has to be considered. Such cases need urgent referral to have this excluded.

Cholesteatoma

This weird-sounding word is used for a very destructive middle ear disorder which is always cause for concern in any ear with active chronic otitis media – not only because of the middle ear destruction but also because it has potential for complications such as mastoiditis and intracranial spread of infection.

Negative middle ear pressure – mentioned above associated with a dysfunctional eustachian tube – causes the eardrum to retract into the middle ear space. Sometimes this retraction process is confined just to one area of the drum and results in the formation of a retraction pocket. The more common sites for these retraction pockets to form are either in the postero-superior portion of the drum between the malleus handle and the posterior margin, or in the pars flaccida portion of the drum. Since the outside layer of the drum is covered by desquamating squamous epithelium, this now forms the lining of the pocket. Problems arise because the normal outward migration of desquamated epithelium no longer operates within these pockets and squamous debris accumulates. See Figure 4.4. The pearly white keratin debris was originally thought to be cholesterol – hence the derivation of the name cholesteatoma. These pockets gradually start behaving like epidermoid cysts and invade the middle ear cleft – particularly upwards into the attic area and backwards into the mastoid antrum (hence the derivation of another name for this condition – attico-antral disease).

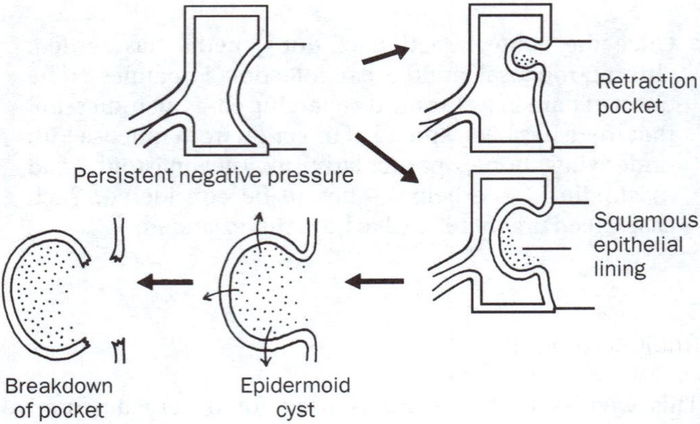

Figure 4.4 Cholesteatoma

If the squamous-lined cholesteatoma 'sac' comes into contact with bone, the bone is eroded away. This bone may be an ossicle (conductive deafness), the facial nerve canal (facial nerve palsy), or the lateral semicircular canal (vertigo).

These cholesteatoma sacs tend to become infected and are one cause of active chronic otitis media. Because the sacs obstruct drainage from the mastoid air cell system, they are a potent cause of mastoiditis and, for some reason, predispose to the intracranial complications of mastoiditis.

Cholesteatoma is a difficult condition to diagnose and even ENT specialists often need to use the operating microscope and microsuction before they can identify cholesteatoma. Clues for the non-specialist are a scanty, smelly discharge, failure to respond to medical treatment, and the presence of pain which may be the first indication of spread of infection to cause mastoiditis.

Any patient with a chronically discharging ear that has not responded to one or two courses of treatment should be referred to exclude cholesteatoma.

The treatment of cholesteatoma is surgical with eradication of the cholesteatoma and an attempt to reconstruct a middle ear sound-conducting mechanism. Sometimes this is possible with what is known as a 'closed' technique but more often disease is eradicated by creating a large mastoid cavity that opens into the ear canal – the radical mastoidectomy.

Mastoiditis

Mastoiditis is the dreaded complication of middle ear cleft infection because it carries a high risk of intracranial spread of infection – meningitis, extradural abscess, sigmoid sinus thrombosis, temporal lobe abscess, cerebellar abscess – see under *Relations of the middle ear*, Chapter 1. Mastoiditis occurs when infection is trapped within the mastoid air cell system and then spreads into the surrounding bone to cause a mastoid osteitis (hence mastoiditis). See Figure 4.5. In children, entrapment is usually caused by the swollen mucosa of an acute otitis media (be suspicious of persisting pain or toxicity in a child with acute otitis media). In adults, this can be the cause but it more often arises from swollen mucosa or a cholesteatoma in active chronic otitis media. As the osteitis develops (pain/tenderness), the soft tissue over the mastoid becomes inflamed and swollen (postauricular swelling). The presence of postauricular swelling usually indicates that a sub-periosteal abscess is forming over the mastoid bone. Remember that intracranial spread of infection may be occurring at the same time (headache, meningism, etc.). See Figure 4.6.

Once mastoiditis is diagnosed, management involves use of high-dose intravenous antibiotics and urgent interventional surgery to decompress the mastoid abscess and eradicate any osteitic bone (cortical mastoidectomy). If cholesteatoma is present a radical mastoidectomy will be needed. Close monitoring is required to detect any intracranial spread of infection at an early stage, in which case neurosurgical intervention is required.

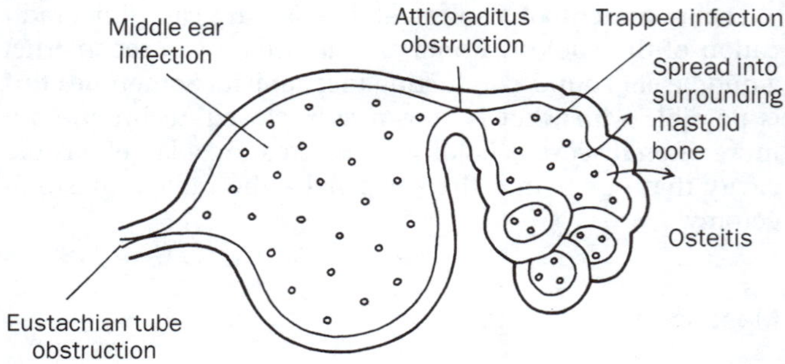

Figure 4.5 Mastoiditis

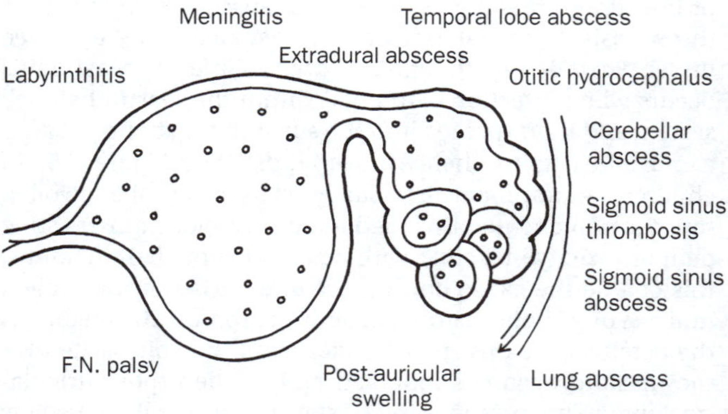

Figure 4.6 Potential complications of mastoiditis

Otosclerosis

In otosclerosis there is an overgrowth of 'spongy' bone in the bony capsule of the inner ear. When this involves the oval window, the stapes becomes fixed and the result is a conductive deafness. It probably has a genetic origin – most common in people of European origin, less common in those of Asian origin, and almost unknown in those of African origin. Presentation is usually in the 20 to 40 age group and in women the process is accelerated by pregnancy. It can be unilateral but tends to be bilateral. The conductive deafness can be managed with a hearing aid but the preferred option is surgical – stapedectomy. In this delicate operation the stapes is removed and replaced by a minute, piston-shaped prosthesis. See Figure 4.7.

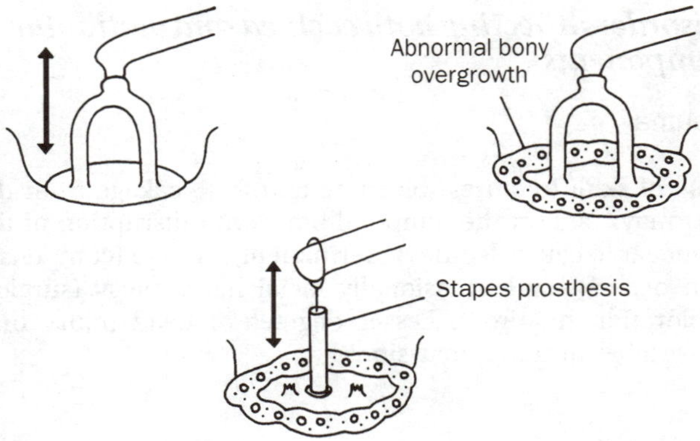

Figure 4.7 Otosclerosis

Unusual middle ear disease

Always consider the possibility of TB when granulation tissue is a prominent feature of a chronic suppurative otitis media. Tuberculous otitis media frequently precipitates a facial nerve palsy. (Remember cholesteatoma may also precipitate a facial palsy.)

> The combination of a discharging ear and a facial palsy is to be regarded as TB until proven otherwise.

Middle ear neoplasia is rare. Benign neoplasia (glomus tumour – a chemodectoma) presents with pulsating tinnitus and an abnormal, reddish tympanic membrane. Malignant neoplasia presents with persistent, severe pain in an ear full of granulation tissue.

The inner ear

Disorders affecting both cochlea and vestibular components

Trauma

Base of skull fractures (bleeding and CSF leakage from the ear) may transect the temporal bone with disruption of the inner ear to cause deafness (permanent), vertigo (compensation occurs), and occasionally facial nerve palsy (surgical exploration required). Lesser degrees of head injury may cause labyrinthine concussion.

Labyrinthitis

Labyrinthitis is uncommon. The complex of spaces and channels within the temporal bone that comprises the inner ear is known as the labyrinth. Infection may spread into the labyrinth either from meningitis – the perilymph of the inner ear is in communication with CSF, **hence the need to be aware of deafness as a complication of meningitis** – or from infection in the middle ear cleft, particularly when cholesteatoma has eroded the bony capsule of the labyrinth. Deafness and vertigo accompany such infection, which usually destroys all the membranes and hair cells of both cochlea and vestibular system to cause a 'dead ear'. Management is by intravenous antibiotics, surgical eradication of middle ear disease, and wide exposure of the labyrinth to allow drainage.

Acoustic neuroma (schwannoma)

Acoustic neuroma is rare. The 8th cranial nerve passes from

the inner ear via the internal auditory canal to the brain stem (cerebellopontine angle), and comprises both auditory and vestibular nerves. A schwannoma may develop on either of these but as it expands will involve both to cause balance disorder (often very non-specific) and a sensorineural deafness. Management is either by stereotactic radiotherapy or by surgical excision.

> Suspect this as the cause in all cases of unilateral sensorineural deafness in adults. Although rare, it does occur in children.

Disorders affecting the cochlea (sensorineural deafness)

Disorders of the cochlea causing sensorineural deafness generally require specialist evaluation. The list of potential causes is included because, among other things, it illustrates the importance of preventive education.

Congenital (genetic). The incidence is about 1:1 000 live births. Consanguinity results in a four-fold increase in the incidence. It may be dominant (family history), recessive (tend to be sporadic), or part of a syndrome (two examples are Waardenburg syndrome – deafness with patchy depigmentation, especially of eyes and the forelock of the hair – and Usher's syndrome – deafness with retinitis pigmentosa).

Congenital (acquired). Rubella is the most important of these causes, hence the importance of immunization of all girls before child-bearing age.

Birth asphyxia. There is a relationship to cerebral palsy, hence the need for good obstetric services.

Neonatal jaundice. The brain-stem auditory pathway is one of those that are damaged should kernicterus develop, hence the need for phototherapy and for blood replacement transfusion when bilirubin levels rise.

The importance of these causes for deafness lies also in the need for early recognition – see *Deafness in children*, Chapter 5, page 74 – in order that rehabilitation may be started before one year of age for optimal speech and intellectual development.

Infantile meningitis. See under *Labyrinthitis*, page 54. The severity of deafness as a complication of meningitis can be reduced by the use of steroids. The two organisms most implicated are Haemophilus and Pneumococcus. It is hoped that the introduction of vaccination may help reduce the prevalence of this complication.

Infectious diseases of childhood. Mumps classically causes unilateral deafness, hence the importance of vaccination.

Ototoxic drugs. These drugs should be available only on prescription from a medical practitioner but in some parts of the world their use is still uncontrolled. Ototoxicity is an important reason for monitoring blood levels during intensive therapy. Salicylate-induced deafness is the only kind that is reversible. Ototoxic drugs include aminoglycoside antibiotics (for example gentamicin, streptomycin), quinine and derivatives, some of the diuretics, and salicylates.

Noise-induced hearing loss. Excessive noise damages hair cells – particularly those towards the basal end of the cochlea – hence the predominant deafness around 4 000 Hz. Noise restriction and noise protection in the work place are important preventive measures.

Syphilis. This is included because it is about the only cause of sensorineural deafness that can be treated (amoxycillin and steroid) if recognized early. Deafness occurs during the early tertiary phase – **be aware of it in adults, particularly in the age range 40 to 60 years, presenting with sudden or rapid onset of either unilateral or bilateral sensorineural deafness.**

Age. Hair cell loss with ageing causes the predominantly high-tone sensorineural hearing loss known as presbyacusis. The disability of deafness adds to the burden of ageing but can often be helped by prescription of suitable hearing aids.

Disorders affecting the vestibular system (vertigo)

Almost all of the disorders of balance that present with vertigo require specialist evaluation. There are several causes for vertigo – see Figure 4.8.

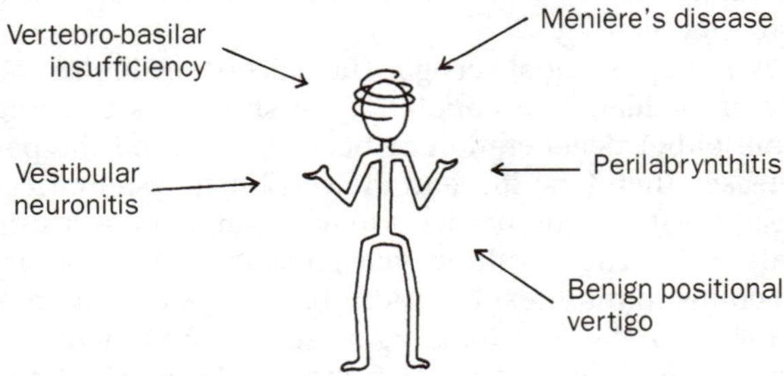

Figure 4.8 Causes for vertigo

Vestibular neuronitis. Neither the precise aetiology nor the pathology are known but the condition is best regarded as a viral neuritis (see also *Bell's palsy*, page 59) that causes either a neuropraxia or nerve degeneration in the vestibular nerve. These patients present initially with acute vertigo requiring bed rest and sedation. This lasts for several days. If there is only neuropraxia, complete resolution should take place over the next few weeks but if there is nerve degeneration, the vestibular system will have to undergo central compensation and this takes several months.

Ménière's disease. Simplistically, this disorder is caused by an increase in the pressure within the endolymphactic compartment of the membranous inner ear. (This may have something to do with osmotic pressure – remember the difference in ionic composition between endolymph and perilymph.) As the pressure increases (endolymphatic hydrops) hair cell stimulation causes tinnitus (cochlea) and vertigo (vestibular) with sustained pressure causing hair cell damage (deafness). Predominantly affecting young to middle-aged adults, it is characterized by episodes that occur in clusters with periods of remission between clusters but steadily deteriorating hearing. The vertigo is managed with 'sea-sickness' preparations and sedatives, and the underlying disorder is treated with salt and caffeine restriction, vasodilators, and diuretics. In severe cases, surgical relief may be contemplated. Options include endolymphatic sac decompression, vestibular nerve section, or inner ear destruction (labyrinthectomy).

Benign positional vertigo. The hairs of vestibular hair cells are embedded in a cupola. These structures can fragment from either degeneration or head trauma and the particles released then float loose in the vestibular system. In certain head positions the particles may impinge on and stimulate hair cells. The resulting vertigo lasts only a short time (seconds to minutes) but tends to recur each time the head returns to the precipitating position. Treatment involves positional manoeuvres to try and get the particles to lodge somewhere out of harm's way.

Perilabyrinthitis/serous labyrinthitis. Middle ear infection, particularly when there has been bone erosion by cholesteatoma, may cause a 'neighbourhood' reaction in the labyrinth, manifesting with vertigo. Surgical exploration is required to eradicate infection.

Vertebro-basilar insufficiency (VBI). The vertebral artery travels through channels in the cervical vertebrae and in the osteo-arthritic spine it may be 'pinched', particularly with head extension. This is a common problem in the middle-aged and elderly, and usually manifests with 'drop attacks' or faintness, but this diminution of blood flow to the vestibular nuclei may cause vertigo. Treatment is with physiotherapy and use of a cervical collar.

Facial nerve palsy

Facial nerve palsy occurs at any age with a prevalence of about 1:5 000 of the population per year. Of these about 80 per cent will be idiopathic (see below).

Upper motor neurone facial palsy occurs as part of a cerebrovascular accident affecting the motor cortex. The diagnosis should be obvious. (Elucidation of 'forehead sparing' can be misleading as often this is the first area to recover in a lower motor neurone facial palsy.)

The most common cause of a lower motor neurone facial palsy is idiopathic and this diagnosis is given the name **Bell's palsy**. The aetiology and precise pathology are unknown but it is most usefully considered as a neuritis which may manifest as either neuropraxia or nerve degeneration. Typically the palsy is of sudden onset and there may be associated otalgia. The palsy may be partial or complete. It is unfortunately a diagnosis that has to be made by excluding all the other potential causes for a facial palsy. This is important because all of these require treatment, whereas an idiopathic palsy is usually left to recover on its own, although many specialists advocate the use of steroids. Full recovery within two to three months occurs with neuropraxia, but when there has been nerve degeneration, recovery is uncertain and may take up to a year.

Herpes zoster oticus is a variation on this disorder in which the causative agent is obvious, since herpes zoster vesicles (shingles) erupt in and around the ear canal indicating involvement of the geniculate ganglion of the facial nerve. This is sometimes known as Ramsay Hunt syndrome. Acyclovir is the current drug of choice.

The other causes for a facial palsy are differentiated by systematic consideration of the facial nerve anatomy; see Figure 4.9.

From the brain stem into the internal auditory canal:

- Trauma with avulsion (rare)
- Meningitis (rare, think of TB)
- Aberrant blood vessels (facial tic or spasm)
- Acoustic neuroma (rare)

Within the temporal bone adjacent to the inner ear:

- Trauma with fracture of the petrous portion of the temporal bone. This requires surgical exploration to either decompress or repair the nerve.

Within the middle ear and mastoid:

- Acute otitis media. This is usually seen in children when the

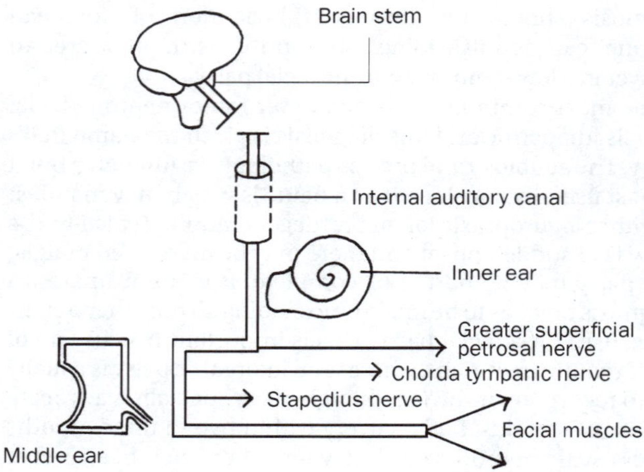

Figure 4.9 Facial nerve anatomy

treatment is IV antibiotics and drainage of the middle ear.

- Chronic otitis media (particularly cholesteatoma but think of TB)
- Mastoiditis
- Trauma with fracture of the mastoid portion of the temporal bone

These require surgical exploration to eradicate disease and to explore the nerve in case repair is needed.

Exit at the stylomastoid foramen into the parotid gland and then distributing to the facial muscles:

- Congenital trauma – within the birth canal the mandibular branch may be compressed (a not uncommon injury), forceps delivery
- Other trauma – penetrating, blunt
- Malignant neoplasm
- Parotitis

As a general rule, facial nerve palsy requires specialist evaluation as a matter of urgency (if such a service is available) for all causes other than idiopathic palsy.

5 A practical approach to ear disorders

Unless they have had it before or have been told what is wrong with their ear, patients don't usually come complaining of a particular disease. They usually come in with a collection of symptoms and expect you to tell them what is wrong. A practical approach to ear disorders is largely based on elucidation of patient symptoms, followed up by examining their ears, since this combination should enable most diagnoses to be made. With external and middle ear disorders you cannot rely on the history/symptoms alone because, although to a certain extent history will help in differentiating between external and middle ear disorders, in the end you are going to have to look in the ear and test the hearing to make the diagnosis. On the other hand, history/symptoms are all-important with inner ear disorders since the only methods of examination are either by audiological evaluation or by radiology. Audiometry is essential when the inner ear disorder affects the cochlea (deafness) but vestibular disorders are predominantly diagnosed from just the history.

In this chapter the different disorders that could potentially be causing the symptoms are discussed. Once a diagnosis has been made, refer to Chapter 4, *Core knowledge of ear disorders,* in which each of the disorders is briefly discussed and guidelines for management of the disorder are given.

Symptoms

Symptoms arising from ear disorders are:

- Otalgia (pain)
- Otorrhoea (discharge)
- Impaired hearing and deafness

- Tinnitus
- Disequilibrium and vertigo
- Facial nerve palsy

Otalgia

Otalgia (pain in the ear) usually arises from inflammation in either the ear canal or the middle ear. The history may provide clues but diagnosis relies largely on examination of the ear. When the appearance of these areas is normal, referred pain has to be considered either from an adjacent structure or one sharing the same innervation as the ear.

Potential causes

The potential causes for otalgia are described below.

External ear

Localized otitis externa – a furuncle. This should be suspected as the cause when there is tenderness on manipulating the pinna or tragal cartilage. Surprisingly, it is easily missed when inserting an otoscope speculum unless the entrance to the ear canal is first inspected.

Later stages of generalized otitis externa. In the early stages the complaint is often merely of an itchy ear, pain starting with the onset of a definite inflammation and swelling of the soft tissues of the ear canal.

Herpes zoster oticus (shingles). This can be a difficult diagnosis to make in the early stages before the vesicular eruption occurs. Since the pain can be intense, the patient may find it strange that you cannot see anything abnormal. The disorder becomes obvious when the vesicles erupt.

Impacted wax or a foreign body in the ear canal. Patients usually experience discomfort rather than pain, unless they have been fiddling in the ear canal and have precipitated an inflammation.

Perichondritis. This is an uncommon, inflammatory swelling of the soft tissues of the pinna that may or may not be associated with an otitis externa. It may also be precipitated by trauma. It requires urgent, vigorous treatment, preferably with intravenous antibiotics, as the infection may spread to involve the cartilage with subsequent deforming contracture (cauliflower ear). Be particularly wary when it occurs in a diabetic or immunocompromised patient as the infection in these patients can rapidly spread into the temporal bone with potentially fatal consequences – necrotizing otitis externa.

Tympanic membrane

Bullous myringitis. This is one of the most painful ear disorders and is probably a viral infection that manifests with small blisters on the eardrum that may contain either serum or blood. It is probably the only indication for using ear drops containing a local anaesthetic.

Middle ear

Acute otitis media. In a typical case this should not be too difficult to diagnose – an irritable child with pyrexia and a sore ear who has an obviously inflamed eardrum. But the symptoms caused by an acute otitis media are very variable, which is why examination of the ears is an essential part of the general examination of an unwell child. Although most common in children, acute otitis media occurs at any age.

Developing mastoiditis. This is included as a separate entity from frank mastoiditis – which is a potential, although uncommon, complication of all middle ear disorders – because it should always be in the back of your mind when there is middle ear infection and otalgia. **In acute otitis media, persistent pain that has not settled once antibiotics have had a chance to work is a 'red flag' symptom**. Chronic otitis media is a painless disorder and the onset of pain is again a 'red flag' symptom. Early mastoiditis often responds to antibiotics alone, whereas established mastoiditis requires mastoid surgery, so that, if suspected, you should refer these patients urgently for a specialist opinion.

Mastoiditis. Once mastoiditis has become established, the diagnosis is much more obvious. The patient is pyrexial and obviously ill, and there is an inflammatory swelling behind the pinna. As mentioned, **mastoiditis is uncommon, but unfortunately it often arises in neglected ears and in such cases intracranial spread of infection may have already occurred by the time the patient comes to see you. You need to be aware of this possibility**.

Middle ear effusion. In children, this disorder is often associated with intermittent discomfort which is probably caused by pressure changes in the middle ear. These children may also present with a painful ear as they seem to be more prone to episodes of acute otitis media than children with normal middle ears.

Barotrauma. Anyone who has flown in an aircraft will be aware that a number of people experience intense pain in their ears during descent. During ascent, as the air pressure in the cabin falls, air from the middle ear passively passes down the eustachian tube to equalize the pressure. However, during descent, as the air pressure rises again, the eustachian tube has to be actively opened either by swallowing or by self-inflation – Valsalva manoeuvre – and not everyone is able to do this, particularly small children. If the pressure in the middle ear cannot be equalized, acute retraction of the eardrum causes intense pain. Similarly, during diving, the middle ear pressure has to be equalized every so often during descent. Persistent negative middle ear pressure may precipitate an acute middle ear effusion and sometimes this is accompanied by bleeding from the middle ear mucosa – haemotympanum.

Referred pain

The ear has a complex sensory innervation which includes, among others, branches from the 5th (trigeminal), 7th (facial), 9th (glossopharyngeal) and 10th (vagus) cranial nerves. These latter two also supply sensory innervation to structures in the aerodigestive tract – it is not uncommon for patients to cough when you fiddle in their ears. Therefore anything irritating or causing inflammation of structures in the oral cavity, pharynx, or larynx may also cause pain to be felt in the ear.

Tonsillitis/pharyngitis and tonsillectomy. It is very easy to assume that otalgia is arising from these disorders but you have to bear in mind that there may be a co-existing otitis media. Always examine the ears to exclude this when otalgia is associated with these disorders.

Dental causes. Erupting teeth, impacted molars, caries, and dental-associated infection are quite common causes for referred pain when the ear is normal on examination.

Temporomandibular joint dysfunction. This is one of the most common causes for referred pain in adults, usually those with dentures. With a full set of natural teeth, no pressure is normally exerted on the articulating surfaces in the temporomandibular joint during mastication, as the upper and lower teeth grind together. When teeth are extracted the alveolar ridge gradually becomes re-absorbed. Dentures may fit well soon after extraction but, after some time, begin to 'overclose' during mastication, exerting pressure on the joint surfaces. This may cause pain which, since the joint is right next to the ear, is experienced as an earache. The management is referral back to the dentist to have the dentures adjusted.

Pharyngeal and laryngeal neoplasia. Look up *The ENT Ten*, page xii, and you will see that this is number 7, a definite 'red flag' symptom. Never forget it, as it may make the difference between referral early enough to offer the patient a reasonable chance of cure and late referral with a poor prognosis.

Cervical osteo-arthritis. A number of people with this disorder – and remember that the process starts in the 40s – have referred otalgia among the other symptoms caused by it.

Treatment

Once a diagnosis of the cause for the otalgia has been made, the appropriate treatment can be initiated (see Chapter 4, *Core knowledge of ear disorders,* and Table 5.1).

Table 5.1 Otalgia

Ear canal:
Furuncle – localized otitis externa
Inflamed/swollen – generalized otitis externa
Normal – examine drum
Eardrum:
Inflamed/bulging – acute otitis media
Blister – bullous myringitis
Dull/retracted – otitis media with effusion
Active perforation – potential complications
Normal – referred pain

Otorrhoea

Otorrhoea (discharge) originates from infection in either the external ear canal or within the middle ear cavity. A history is helpful but diagnosis relies largely on examination of the ear. Discharge from otitis externa is usually scanty and initially associated with itching or discomfort. The middle ear is mucosal lined and the discharge of chronic infection is usually both mucoid and profuse although cholesteatomatous disease may produce only a scanty, smelly discharge. Acute otitis media usually presents with otalgia, which is often relieved when the drum perforates to produce a discharge. Discharges also include bleeding and this is usually related to trauma, either local within the ear canal or from fractures of the base of skull.

Potential causes

The potential causes of otorrhoea are described below.

External ear

Otitis externa. The localized form is a furuncle in the hair-bearing area which, when it points and bursts, will discharge blood-stained pus. The generalized form is an inflammation of the ear canal skin. When this weeps it will produce a pus discharge into an ear canal which is often full of debris-containing desquamated epithelium and wax. With some fungal infections the appearance of the debris has been likened to wet newspaper.

Middle ear

Acute otitis media after perforation. Typically there will have been a pyrexial illness with a sore ear which then 'bursts' to discharge blood-stained mucopus. Surprisingly, in infants not all of the precipitating episodes of otitis media seem to be particularly painful.

Active chronic otitis media. In this case, ears known to have a perforation will begin to discharge either after an episode of upper respiratory tract infection or after water has got into the ear. The discharge is usually profuse and mucopurulent. Many patients with this disorder seem to be particularly neglectful of their ears and the discharge may have been going on for quite some time before they seek medical attention. If the discharge is particularly malodorous, suspect underlying cholesteatoma. Cholesteatoma should also be suspected when the infection fails to respond to treatment.

Previous mastoid surgery and an infected cavity. Scars behind the ear will indicate that either mastoid surgery or reconstructive middle ear surgery (tympanoplasty) has been performed – it is surprising how many patients do not know what type of surgery they have had! It is easy to overlook a mastoid cavity when examining the ear unless the posterior wall of the ear canal is specifically examined. Wax commonly accumulates in these cavities and they are often the site of chronic infection.

Ear trauma and head injury

Bleeding is indicative of either local trauma in the canal, perforation of the tympanic membrane, or a fracture of the base of the skull. This latter is often associated with a CSF leak which creates a 'halo' sign on the ear dressing.

Blood-staining on the cotton wool used to dry mop a discharging ear (see Chapter 14, page 187) usually arises from granulation tissue associated with prolonged infection.

Treatment

Once the cause for otorrhoea has been established, the appropriate treatment can be initiated (see Chapter 4, *Core knowledge of ear disorders,* and Table 5.2).

Table 5.2 Otorrhoea

Ear canal:
Furuncle – localized otitis externa
Inflamed/swollen – generalized otitis externa
mastoid cavity – infected mastoid cavity
Normal – examine eardrum
Eardrum:
Short history/fresh perforation – acute otitis media
Longer history/active perforation – active chronic otitis media
Fleshy polyp – active chronic otitis media (cholesteatoma)

Impaired hearing and deafness

Deafness in children is a special topic and will be dealt with next.

Note that the terms 'hearing impairment' and 'deafness' are not strictly synonymous although they are used very loosely. A hearing impairment should refer to mild/moderate hearing loss and deafness to severe/profound hearing loss.

When a patient presents with deafness you want to know not only the cause of the deafness but also the degree of handicap experienced because this may be a determinant factor in management. Not all patients with deafness want or warrant surgery or hearing aids. Potential causes are listed below, some with characteristic features in the history, others with characteristic examination findings or audiometry. It is useful to remember to ask in what situations they experience difficulty as often patients with a conductive deafness are less handicapped in noisy environments (they don't hear the background noise and people tend to speak louder in such situations), whereas it is the opposite for patients with a sensorineural deafness.

Examination of the ear should reveal most of the causes for conductive deafness. Response to voice testing should give you some idea as to the degree of hearing loss, and you should determine whether the deafness is a conductive or a sensorineural loss (response to tuning fork testing). Once deafness is confirmed, referral for audiological evaluation and specialist management is required.

Potential causes

The potential causes described below cover all three parts of the ear.

External ear

Impacted wax or foreign body. These problems will only cause deafness when the entire ear canal is obstructed. The deafness should be relieved when the wax or foreign body is removed.

Occlusion by swelling – infection. Again, deafness is noticed only when the canal is obstructed by either the swelling or the discharge/debris accumulation. Once the disorder has been treated and has resolved, the deafness should be relieved.

Congenital or acquired stenosis. Not all deformed pinnas are associated with complete stenosis of the canal and conversely there may be a complete canal stenosis with a normal pinna.

Tympanic membrane

Perforation. The degree of hearing impairment usually relates to the size of the perforation. This is not always the case, however, as there may be middle ear adhesions or disruptions of the ossicular chain as part of whatever caused the perforation.

Tympanosclerosis with middle ear involvement. The process causing tympanosclerosis in the eardrum (chalk patches) may also extend to involve the middle ear mucosa and impinge on the ossicular chain.

Scarring with middle ear adhesions. Scarring is indicative of healed otitis media and there may be adhesions or disruption of the ossicular chain as well.

Middle ear

Middle ear effusion. This is the most common cause of hearing impairment in children – otitis media with effusion – but it does occur at any age after an episode of otitis media. In adults, it may be associated with barotrauma, usually after flying in an aircraft.

> When the effusion is unilateral, especially in adults, pathology in the nasopharynx always has to be excluded.

Active chronic otitis media. There are several causes for deafness in this disorder – the perforation, mucopus in the middle ear, inflammatory swelling of mucosa around the ossicles, or osteitis causing ossicular chain disruption. When the underlying cause is cholesteatoma, this disease destroys the ossicles.

Inactive chronic otitis media. Here again the deafness may arise from the perforation or the end result of middle ear disease – adhesions or disruption of the ossicular chain.

Ossicular chain discontinuity. Infection and cholesteatoma have been mentioned earlier, but trauma may also be a cause.

Ossicular chain fixation. Tympanosclerosis and fibrosis have been mentioned earlier, but consider otosclerosis as well.

Inner ear

Congenital. The usual classifications of congenital disorders apply also to deafness. Genetic causes may be familial or sporadic, dominant or recessive, syndromic or non-syndromic. Congenital deafness may be the result of a disorder in utero (acquired), of which the most common disease is rubella.

Natal causes usually relate to asphyxia or intracerebral haemorrhage. Children who have experienced these disorders usually have some degree of cerebral palsy or retardation.

Neonatal. The neonatal disorder that causes deafness is kernicterus. However, when neonates require admission to neonatal intensive care units they are exposed to a variety of causes for deafness, apart from their underlying illness, of which the most likely cause is ototoxic drugs. All survivors of neonatal intensive care should be regarded as being at risk for deafness and their hearing should be assessed as soon as possible after discharge from the intensive care unit.

Infection. Meningitis is the most likely infection to cause deafness. Mumps classically causes a unilateral deafness. Never forget the possibility of syphilis as a cause for a recent-onset sensorineural deafness in an adult as it is the only one in which the deafness may recover after treatment if it is initiated promptly. The deafness usually comes on fairly suddenly, some 20 to 30 years after the infection was acquired.

Noise exposure. This is diagnosed from the typical 'dip' in the audiogram at 4 000 Hz.

Ototoxic drugs. Salicylate-induced deafness is reversible when the drug is stopped, but the others – aminoglycosides, quinine, cytotoxics – are not.

Ménière's disease. Deafness is one of the triad of symptoms – vertigo, tinnitus, deafness – that characterize this disorder, but the deafness does not always recover after each episode so that there will be a progressive sensorineural deafness.

Trauma. Disruption of middle ear structures has been mentioned earlier. The inner ear may be disrupted when base of skull fractures involve the temporal bone. The deafness does not usually recover. There is also a state known as 'inner ear concussion' when there is no demonstrable fracture, from which recovery may occur.

Tumour – acoustic neuroma. Although rare, this is one disorder otologists always consider when there is a unilateral sensorineural deafness because, if untreated, the tumour will eventually expand and compress the brain stem with fatal consequences.

Age – presbyacusis. This is by far the most common cause for sensorineural deafness and affects a large proportion of any ageing population. Typically, the deafness is bilateral and on audiogram will be seen to predominantly affect the higher tones.

Treatment

Once the diagnosis of the cause of deafness has been determined and the degree of handicap evaluated appropriate management can be initiated.

Surgery. Conductive losses are often corrected with appropriate surgery, for example placement of ventilation tubes for middle ear effusions, or tympanoplasty with or without ossiculoplasty for inactive chronic otitis media. This is not always possible. For example, surgery for cholesteatoma is often destructive rather than reconstructive (radical mastoidectomy), and congenital deformities may not be amenable to surgery and hearing aids may need to be fitted as well as, or instead of, surgery.

Hearing aids. There are also many patients with conductive losses who do not want surgery and would prefer to use a hearing aid. In practice, patients with conductive losses generally derive greater benefit from a hearing aid than patients with sensorineural losses, since their problem is simply one requiring amplification and they do not have the element of distortion that often accompanies sensorineural deafness.

When the handicap of deafness is due to a sensorineural loss, hearing aids are needed. A wide range of hearing aids are available – body-worn aids, postaural aids, in the ear canal aids, spectacle aids. Many sophisticated devices may be built into a hearing aid to make it better able to overcome a specific handicap, such as high-tone or low-tone cut-off, high-tone or low-tone gain, or to make them more acceptable and easier to use, such as directional microphones, automatic cut-off when the sound level exceeds a certain threshold. Of course the cost factor has to be considered – the more sophisticated the aid, the more expensive it will be.

Provision of a hearing aid should be backed up by audiotherapy which teaches the deaf patient all the added 'tricks' to overcome the handicap – making use of lip reading and body language are examples. This is particularly important when the deafness is in the severe to profound range, when even a powerful hearing aid does not restore the hearing threshold to anything like normal.

Cochlear implant. When the deafness is total or near total, the patient may be a candidate for a cochlear implant. This is a very sophisticated device that converts sound into an electrical stimulus which is applied to the auditory nerve via an electrode implanted into the cochlea.

R Often diagnosis of a specific cause for deafness requires specialist expertise. Decisions regarding surgery or prescription and provision of appropriate hearing aids fall largely into the realm of ENT and audiological specialists. However, primary care practitioners need to be aware of what is available and when and where to direct their patients with a deafness problem or to counsel them when they are uncertain as to aspects of their problem.

Deafness in children

Normal hearing is a fundamental requirement for the development of speech in infancy since speech develops as a mimic of sounds heard – if you want to know what type of sounds deaf people are hearing, listen to their speech – it tells you how they are hearing your speech. Hearing impairment causes both delay in speech development and distortion of the quality of the speech that does develop. A more severe degree of deafness results in no speech development at all (deaf and dumb). There is a limited time span in children's development for optimum acquisition of speech and if they are not speaking by the age of five to six years it is unlikely that they will develop intelligible speech thereafter. Hearing is essential for the acquisition of vocabulary since we learn the words first and then give them meaning. Vocabulary is the basis for all learning and, because we think in words, for intellectual development as well. Since speech and hearing are the most rapid forms of communication, the ability to communicate will be impaired by deafness.

For all of these reasons it is essential that deafness in an infant is detected as early as possible, preferably before one year of age, in order that a rehabilitation programme can be commenced to aid speech and intellectual development.

> As a general rule, parents will become aware of hearing problems in their baby early on and it is essential that their opinions are heeded (not ignored or brushed aside) and that these infants are referred for evaluation.

Potential causes

Apart from congenital causes, other infants likely to have hearing problems are those with ear or craniofacial deformities, those who have had meningitis, and those who have required intensive care – the 'high-risk register' for infant deafness.

Testing of hearing in babies and infants is a highly specialized skill and in primary care it is best to question parents to gain an idea as to whether or not there is a hearing impairment. See Table 5.3.

Table 5.3 Questions for use in assessing hearing in babies

Baby only a few weeks old:
Does your baby appear to be listening to you when you talk or sing?
Does your baby open his or her eyes or blink when there is a noise?

Baby about six months old:
Does your baby enjoy you talking or playing word games with him or her?
Does your baby try to see where a noise is coming from by turning his or her eyes or head towards the sound?

Baby about nine months old:
Does your baby appear to enjoy babbling and making other noises?
Does your baby appear to respond to even very soft sounds?

Baby about a year old:
Is your baby beginning to say baby words?
Does your baby respond when you say his or her name and the names of things he or she plays with?

Baby about a year and a half old:
Is your baby beginning to use simple words?
Does your baby pick up or point to things around the house when you ask him or her to do this?

Babies of two years or more:
Is your baby putting words together and trying to talk to you?
Do you think your baby can hear normally even when you speak to him or her in a very soft voice?

Treatment

In childhood, conductive causes for hearing impairment are common, particularly middle ear effusions. At this level of hearing loss there is not the same urgency but a persistent loss over several months will begin to impair speech quality, vocabulary progression and intellectual development. Behaviour problems frequently accompany middle ear effusions and these children are often clumsy. These children need referral for assessment as not only are conductive losses remediable with surgery, for example ventilation tubes, but sometimes a sensorineural hearing loss is mistaken for a conductive loss and in these cases provision of hearing aids may be more appropriate.

Tinnitus

Tinnitus is a subjective ringing or buzzing sound in the ear. To understand tinnitus, think of the auditory system as simply a hair cell with a neurone connecting it to the auditory centre – see Figure 5.1. Any impulse generated in the neurone in such a system will be interpreted by the auditory centre as a sound. Normally such an impulse is only generated by the hair cell in response to external sounds transmitted via the ear canal, middle ear, and cochlea. Tinnitus arises when impulses are generated by other mechanisms.

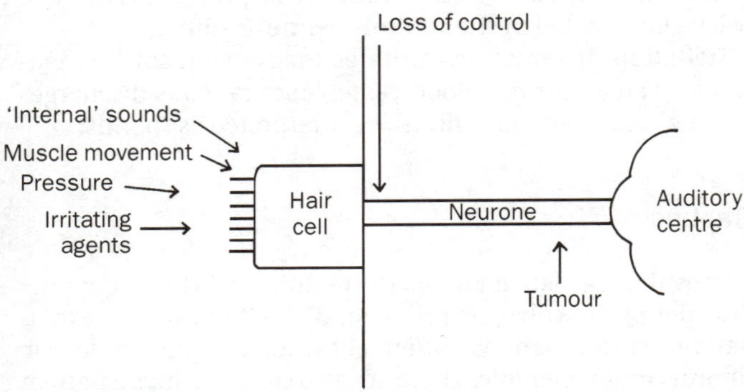

Figure 5.1 Tinnitus

Potential causes

The approach to tinnitus involves detection of any of the causes described below from the history and examination. This should be supplemented by audiological investigation to detect any deafness associated with either hair cell loss or neurone impairment. Possible causes are:

Stimulation of the hair cell. This may be internal sounds not normally heard, such as vascular pulsations in the carotid artery or in a vascular middle ear tumour, or it could be from movement of muscles in the middle ear, such as the tensor tympani muscle which attaches to the malleus.

Other types of stimulation. Sometimes an inner ear disorder may stimulate the hair cell by some mechanism other than sound vibration. The pressure changes in the inner ear fluids that occur in Ménières disease can do this, as can irritative disorders such as labyrinthitis, ototoxics (particularly salicylates), or sensitivity to stimulants such as caffeine.

Damaged hair cell. Neurones connected to sensory organs are spontaneously excitable – by this we mean that they are capable of producing spontaneous, but random, action potentials. Normally the rate at which these are produced is controlled by the sensory organ. In the cochlea this is the hair cell. If the hair cell is damaged (noise trauma, ototoxics) or lost (ageing) these now uncontrolled spontaneous action potentials – impulses – will continue to be produced and each will be interpreted by the auditory centre as sound.

Irritation. If something irritates the nerve (acoustic neuroma or an abnormal blood vessel) spontaneous discharges may be generated that will also be interpreted as sounds.

Treatment

Removal of causative factors or treatment of the underlying disorder may resolve the problem. When it doesn't, an explanation to the patient will often relieve anxiety and render the tinnitus more tolerable. There are also simple things a patient can do that may help. Tinnitus tends to be masked by external noise (which is why it is usually worse in quiet surroundings) so that having music playing or a radio on is often helpful (sleep buttons on clock radios). Provision of a hearing aid is a way of increasing the external sound input when tinnitus is a complication of deafness. Sophisticated masking devices based on hearing aids are available for really troublesome tinnitus. Where a tinnitus clinic exists, this is a useful resource for referral.

Disequilibrium and vertigo

The brain-stem vestibular centres co-ordinate input into the balance system from the vestibular organs in the two ears, from the eyes, and from joints and muscles in the cervical spine and the limbs. The cerebellum then co-ordinates body movements in response to these sensory inputs. The cerebrum probably exerts some overall control but is primarily where awareness of balance is centred, the sensation of disequilibrium resulting from a faulty or contradictory input from one or more of the sensory input systems.

Classically, symptoms are divided into either true vertigo (a sensation of rotation or movement often accompanied

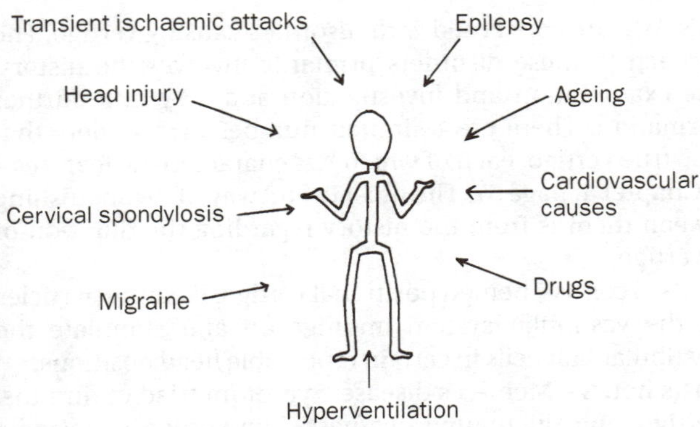

Figure 5.2 Causes for dizziness

by nausea) or other symptoms such as lightheadedness (a feeling of fainting), unsteadiness or imbalance (a tendency to fall or veer to one side), and blackouts. This division is made because these other symptoms result from disorders such as hypotension, cardiac arrhythmias, epilepsy, other neurological disorders, and the ageing process with its gradual deterioration in co-ordination (see Figure 5.2), whereas vertigo is usually caused by vestibular disorders (see Figure 5.3).

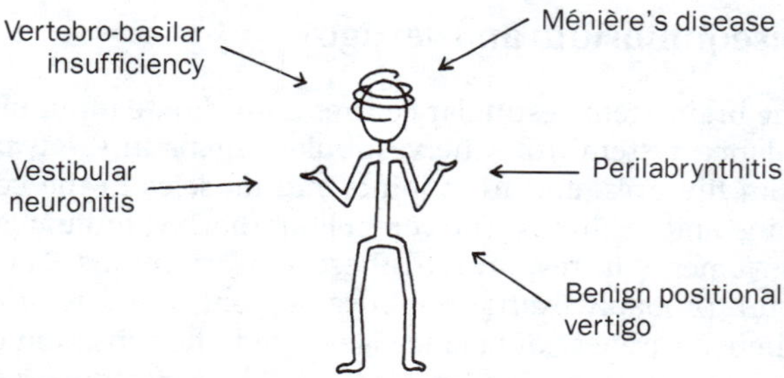

Figure 5.3 Causes for vertigo

Potential causes

In ENT we are concerned with disorders causing vertigo. The approach to these disorders primarily involves the history, since examination and investigation add very little further information. There are a limited number of disorders that cause true vertigo, each of which has characteristic features – see Chapter 4, page 57. The most useful way of distinguishing between them is from the history regarding the duration of the vertigo.

- Lasts seconds – benign positional vertigo. Floating particles in the vestibular system impinge on and stimulate the vestibular hair cells in certain repeatable head positions.
- Lasts hours – Ménières disease. Symptom triad of tinnitus, vertigo, and fluctuating deafness. The vertigo is episodic and the episodes typically occur in clusters with periods of

remission in between when deafness may recover to some extent.

- Lasts days – vestibular neuronitis. This disorder is probably a viral neuritis affecting one of the vestibular nerves which, by interfering with input into the balance system from one vestibular organ, precipitates acute onset of vertigo which then only gradually settles.

Vertebro-basilar insufficiency. This is caused by cervical osteo-arthritis and interruption of vertebral artery blood flow during cervical spine movements. It is diagnosed from the history regarding the effects of head extension or rotation in precipitating the vertigo.

Concomitant middle ear disease. Examination is most beneficial in detection or exclusion of concomitant middle ear disease that may be the cause for the vertigo:

- Effusions often cause clumsiness and unsteadiness.
- Active chronic otitis media can precipitate a 'neighbourhood' perilabyrinthitis. When this is the cause, it is often because cholesteatoma has eroded the bony capsule of the lateral semicircular canal to expose the membranous labyrinth to the effects of inflammation and infection in the middle ear.

Always think to exclude acoustic neuroma when disequilibrium/vertigo is associated with unilateral deafness and tinnitus.

As far as investigations are concerned, 'positional testing' may aid the diagnosis of cervical osteo-arthritis or benign positional vertigo; audiometry may provide clues in Ménières disease and acoustic neuroma and caloric testing may identify the affected nerve in vestibular neuronitis.

Treatment

Having arrived at a provisional diagnosis, the vertigo will need treatment and the most beneficial is a combination of sea-sickness preparations, sedation, and bed rest. Thereafter

R these patients will usually require specialist referral for evaluation and further management.

Facial nerve palsy

Upper motor neurone facial palsy occurs as part of a cerebrovascular accident affecting the motor cortex and the diagnosis should be obvious. Elucidation of 'forehead sparing' on its own can be misleading as often this is the first area to recover in a lower motor neurone facial palsy.

Potential causes

The most common cause of a lower motor neurone facial palsy is idiopathic and this diagnosis is given the name 'Bell's palsy'. It is unfortunately a diagnosis that can only be made by excluding all the other potential causes for a facial nerve palsy. Apart from diagnosing idiopathic facial palsy, it is important to do this because all of these other causes of facial nerve palsy require treatment, whereas an idiopathic palsy is usually left to recover on its own. Many specialists, however, advocate the use of steroids.

The other causes are differentiated by systematic consideration of the facial nerve anatomy – see Chapter 4, page 60. Clinically, take a history concerning possible recent head trauma, past ear disorder, current otalgia, deafness, tinnitus, or otorrhoea and then examine the ear and the parotid gland. R All of these other causes for facial palsy require ENT specialist referral.

Treatment

Having excluded these disorders and arrived at a diagnosis of Bell's palsy (most usefully considered to be a viral neuritis causing either neuropraxia or nerve degeneration) further consideration is necessary. Clinically, the palsy may be incomplete or complete. Incomplete palsies are indicative of neuropraxia and all recover within a month or two. Complete palsies may result from either neuropraxia or nerve degeneration. In this situation specialist referral is needed in order to distinguish between these states. This is done by observing the response to simple nerve stimulation and comparing the threshold stimulation required to elicit a muscle twitch in both the affected nerve and the nerve on the unaffected side. If both thresholds are similar, then the nerve is in a state of neuropraxia and will recover within two to three months. If there is no muscle twitch response from the affected nerve to the highest tolerated stimulus, the nerve has undergone nerve degeneration. When this is the case, only 50 per cent of such patients will regain an acceptable recovery of facial movement, and this will take 6 to 12 months.

For those patients who do not regain acceptable facial movement, cosmetic surgery (face lift) may help. Eye closure is a problem with exposure keratitis as a complication. In this situation the eyelids have to be partially sutured together to protect the cornea. Sometimes nerve anastomosis is considered. Cross-face nerve grafts from the normally functioning facial nerve on the opposite side or hypoglossal-facial nerve anastomosis are the current options.

PART II
The nose and sinuses

6 Structure and function of the nose and sinuses

ENT surgeons consider the nose in three parts – the external nose, the nasal cavities and associated sinuses, and the post-nasal space. See Figure 6.1.

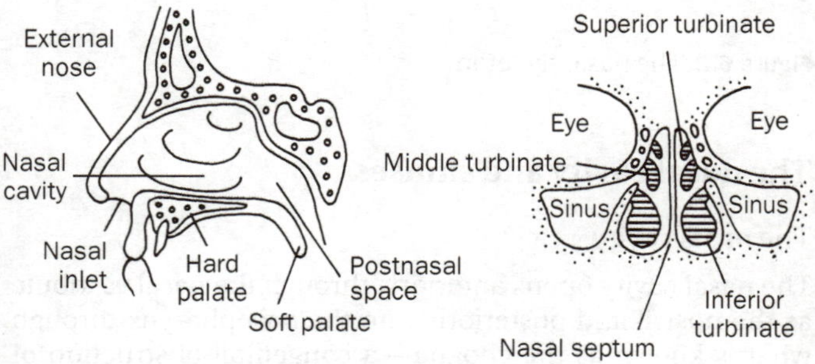

Figure 6.1 The three parts of the nose

The external nose

The external nose forms a cosmetically significant feature of the human face. The upper portion is supported by the nasal bones projecting from the facial skeleton. The lower portion has a cartilaginous skeleton made up of the alar cartilage and the upper lateral cartilage, and relies for forward projection on the integrity of the nasal septal cartilage whose dorsal free margin acts rather like a tent ridgepole. See Figure 6.2. Adjustments to both elements of the skeleton form the basis of cosmetic rhinoplasty surgery. The skin over the cartilaginous skeleton is rather adherent and contains sebaceous glands. These glands may hypertrophy in old age and the resulting cosmetic deformity is known as a rhinophyma.

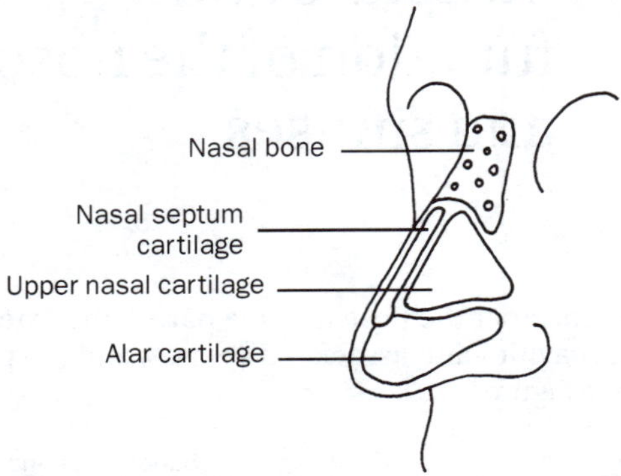

Figure 6.2 The nasal skeleton

The nasal cavity and sinuses

The nasal cavity

The nasal cavity opens anteriorly through the nasal vestibule as the nostril and posteriorly into the nasopharynx through what is known as the choana – a congenital obstruction of this opening is known as choanal atresia. The nasopharynx is also known as the postnasal space and is the space above the soft palate which contains the adenoid and the openings of the eustachian tubes. The two nasal vestibules are lined by hair-bearing skin – the hairs are known as vibrissae – and are separated by the columella. The columella forms the front end of the nasal septum and the septum separates the two nasal cavities. The nasal cavities are lined by ciliated respiratory mucosa in which there are mucus-secreting glands which can produce up to 750 ml of mucus daily. The mucus blanket has both protective and cleansing functions and is continually wafted posteriorly by the action of the cilia, where it will eventually be swallowed. Increased mucus production may become noticeable as a postnasal drip.

The **nasal septum** has a cartilaginous skeleton anteriorly and a bony skeleton posteriorly. It is covered by adherent mucosa in which, anteriorly, there are prominent blood vessels. This vascular area is known as Little's area and is a common site for nose bleeds – see *Cauterizing a nose* in Chapter 14. The septum is often deviated into one or both nostrils either as a result of trauma or because of overgrowth during development. If you think about it, if it grows vertically beyond its anatomical confines it can only be accommodated by buckling into either a C- or S-shape. Therefore, if you are going to straighten the nasal septum, an operation known as septoplasty, you will have to both straighten the cartilage and reduce it in size as well – see Figure 8.3, page 108.

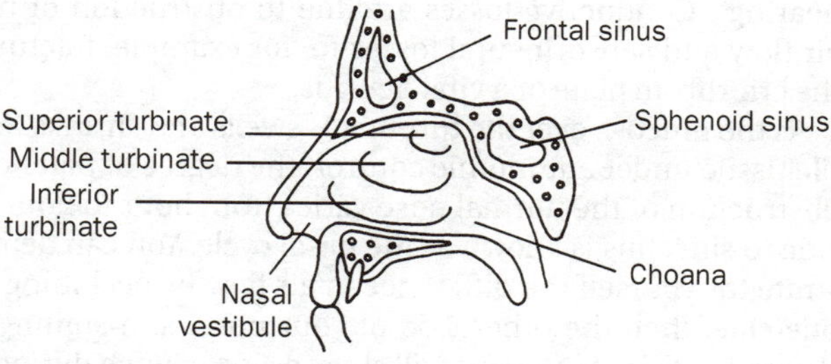

Figure 6.3 Lateral wall of nasal cavity

The lateral wall of the nasal cavity (see Figure 6.3) consists of three bony projections known as turbinates or conchae, covered by lax mucosa beneath which there is a vascular plexus which acts rather like erectile tissue under autonomic control. Sympathetic stimulation of the turbinates causes vasoconstriction and parasympathetic stimulation causes vasodilatation. The turbinates increase the surface area for the 'air-conditioning' function of the nose – warming and humidification of air. The inferior is the largest of the three turbinates, it is about the size of the little finger, and can be seen when examining the nose anteriorly. It can also be seen when examining the postnasal space with a mirror. The other turbinates are smaller but sometimes the middle turbinate can be seen above and behind the anterior end of the inferior turbinate. The spaces beneath the turbinates are known as the meati, of which the most significant is the middle meatus because into this space open many of the sinus drainage channels, known as ostia. The nasolacrimal duct opens anteriorly into the inferior meatus.

The olfactory epithelium is situated above the superior turbinate in the roof of the nose and cannot be seen without special instrumentation (nasal endoscopy). Olfaction, the ability to smell things, depends on scent-laden particles going into solution on the olfactory epithelium. The mechanism of stimulation of the olfactory nerve (1st cranial nerve) is largely unknown. We can, in the clinical situation, consider conductive and sensorineural loss of smell, or anosmia (cf. hearing). Conductive losses are due to obstruction of nasal air flow and sensorineural losses to, for example, fracture of the cribriform plate or a viral neuritis.

As the mucosa over the turbinates swells and shrinks (erectile tissue under autonomic control) the degree of patency or obstruction of the normal nose varies from hour to hour and side to side, this is known as the nasal cycle. You can demonstrate for yourself the difference in air flow by occluding first one side, then the other side of your nose, and sniffing up. Repeating this at intervals will show a side change during the course of the day. The exact reason for this circadian rhythm is obscure, but when it is exaggerated it becomes noticeable and patients may complain about it. In these cases it is often stress that is the perverter of sympathetic/parasympathetic harmony, since a feeling of 'well-being' is dependent on impeccable autonomic balance.

The sinuses

Much of the facial skeleton is hollowed out by air-containing cavities. These are the paranasal sinuses – maxillary, frontal, ethmoidal, and sphenoidal (see Figure 6.4). The most posterior of these is the sphenoidal sinus which opens into the back of the nasal cavity above the choana. The others open into the nasal cavity in the middle meatus beneath the middle turbinate, having rather complex drainage channels (hence this area is known as the ostiomeatal complex). The ostium of the maxillary sinus (maxillary antrum) is situated high up on its medial wall, the ethmoidal sinuses (a complex of air cells between the nasal cavity and the orbit) drain from one into another before opening into the meatus, and the frontal sinus has a long frontonasal duct. This complexity, together with the narrowness of the middle meatus (which can be rendered even more so by minor anatomical abnormalities in this area), predisposes to the obstruction of the sinus ostia which precipitates sinusitis.

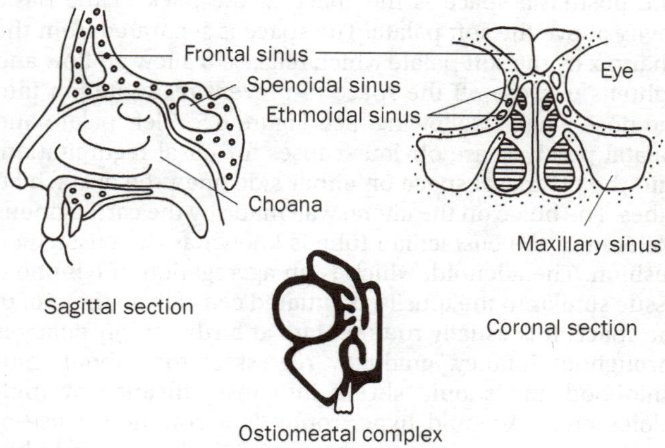

Figure 6.4 The sinuses

The function of the air-containing paranasal sinuses is uncertain since they are not actively involved in respiration. Suggestions have included that they lighten the skull, resonate the voice, strengthen the facial skeleton, and act as shock absorbers for violent blows.

The sinuses have anatomical relations that are important where spread of infection or other disease is concerned:

- Maxillary sinus – orbit, infra-orbital nerve, teeth, nasal cavity, cheek
- Ethmoidal sinuses – orbit (lamina papyracea), anterior cranial fossa (cribriform plate), lacrimal sac, nasal cavity
- Frontal sinus – orbit, anterior cranial fossa, sagittal sinus
- Sphenoidal sinus – internal carotid artery, optic nerve, cavernous sinus (containing the 3rd, 4th, and 6th cranial nerves) and the 1st and 2nd divisions of the 5th cranial nerve.

The postnasal space

The postnasal space is the space at the back of the nasal cavity above the soft palate. The space is separated from the pharynx by the soft palate which relaxes to allow air flow and tightens to close off the space to prevent regurgitation into the nose when swallowing. See Figure 6.5. Cleft palate and palatal paralysis are obvious causes for nasal regurgitation. Into the postnasal space on either side open the eustachian tubes. The bulge on the lateral wall made by the cartilaginous skeleton of the eustachian tube is known as the eustachian cushion. The adenoid, which is an aggregation of lymphoid tissue similar to the tonsils, is situated centrally in the roof of the space. It is usually rudimentary at birth, rapidly enlarges throughout infancy, gradually regresses from about mid-childhood and should shrink into insignificance by mid-adolescence. Adenoid hypertrophy is a common cause of snoring and upper airway obstruction in infants and children, and may predispose to middle ear problems as it interferes with eustachian tube function. For some as yet undetermined reason, a combination of Epstein Barr virus colonization of adenoid tissue remnants, a co-carcinogen, and a genetic susceptibility predispose to formation of a carcinoma in the postnasal space and, since this is a hidden area, the first presentation of a carcinoma may be a metastatic neck node.

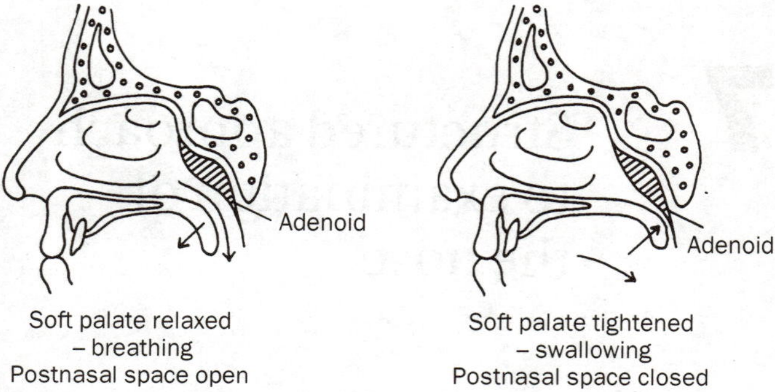

Figure 6.5 Soft palate opening and closing the postnasal space

In summary, the nose has the following functions:

- A respiratory conduit. Note that the neonate appears not to be able to open the mouth to breathe and if the nasal passage is obstructed (for example choanal atresia) will die unless an oral airway is inserted. This life and death matter puts this function at the top of the list.
- An air conditioner (warms, cleans, and humidifies air).
- A reflex organ (sneezing).
- A phonatory resonator. Pinch your nose closed and then start talking – the intelligibility of speech is markedly decreased by the loss of vocal resonance.
- An olfactory organ.

7 Structured approach to examination of the nose

The summary in Table 7.1 will provide you with a basis for examining the nose.

Table 7.1 Aids to examination in rhinology

The external nose

Is the external nose normal? If not, is there an abnormality of:

- The upper bony portion?
- The lower cartilaginous portion?
- The nasal tip, alar cartilages, and central columella?

The nasal cavities

Trying to determine what you are seeing when you start looking into a nasal cavity is a skill that is a little difficult to master. It helps to try to be dogmatic.

Ask yourself first if the available space in the lumen of each nostril is both adequate and symmetrical as you ask the patient to 'sniff in'. If it is not, then what is impinging on the space?

Lateral impingements

- Collapse or deformity of the supporting alar cartilages
- Collapse of a nasal valve
  - soft, floppy alar cartilage
  - external compression
- Enlargement of the inferior turbinate:
  - 'normal'
  - allergic
  - non-allergic

Table 7.1 continued
Medial impingements • Symmetrical: some type of swelling of the anterior end of the nasal septum: – septal haematoma – septal abscess • Asymmetrical: septal deviation **Impingements in the middle of the space** • Foreign body • Nasal polyp • Tumour: – benign – malignant

Step 1

Start with a general examination of the face from the front, focus in on the nose; view the profile from the side, focus in on the nose; view from above, focus in on the nose.

- Does the nose look 'normal' in relation to the rest of the face?
- If not, what is wrong about it?

Answer this question by examining each component to the nose individually.

A. Shield the lower cartilaginous portion and examine the upper bony portion from the front and from the side.

Are the nasal bones any of the following?

- Straight – normal
- Deviated – consider nasal trauma
- Depressed:
  - centrally – consider congenital causes, nasal trauma, tertiary syphilis
  - on one side – consider nasal trauma

- 'Humped' – consider congenital causes, growth characteristics, 'tumours'

B. Shield the upper bony portion and examine the lower cartilaginous portion from the front and from the side.

The dorsal free margin of the cartilaginous septum forms the central ridge. Is this any of the following?
- Straight – normal
- Deviated – consider deviated nasal septum
- Depressed – consider late complications of either septal surgery or septal haematoma/abscess

C. Tilt the head backwards and examine the nasal tip, the alar cartilages, and the columella.

Is the tip any of the following?
- 'Normally rounded' – normal
- Enlarged and bulbous – consider rhinophyma
- Notched – consider congenital causes
- 'Droopy' – consider congenital causes, loss of support with ageing

Are the alar cartilages any of the following?
- Symmetrical – normal
- Offering good support to the nasal vestibule
- Asymmetrical:
  - Is this because one or both are deformed? Consider cleft lip/palate, other congenital causes, trauma, underlying 'tumour'

Is the columella any of the following?
- Straight and reasonably thin – normal
- Deviated – consider deviated nasal septum (push the skin of the columella to one side or the other and you will see the end of the septal cartilage beneath), cleft lip/palate, other congenital causes, trauma
- Abnormally thickened – consider deviated nasal septum, inflammatory swelling, congenital causes

Step 2

While the head is still tilted backwards, push the tip upwards a little with your finger and look a little further into the nasal inlet. After an initial look, request the patient to forcibly 'sniff in' while you are still looking to see what effect this has.

- Is the visible airway symmetrical on both sides?
- If not, you have to determine what is impinging into the visible space to create the asymmetry. Is it something from the lateral wall, something from the medial wall, or something in the centre? Is this asymmetry the result of anything that you have already identified or is it because there is something a little further back impinging into one or both airways? (This area will be examined next.)
- Does this visible airway space markedly narrow during forcible sniffing in – consider loss of support to what is called the 'nasal valve area' by the alar cartilages.

Step 3

Return the head to the upright position. Using a light and some form of nasal speculum, examine into the nasal cavity for as far back as you can see. While doing this you should be looking for secretions/discharges, assessing the status of the mucosa, and attempting to identify firstly normal structures and secondly abnormal masses. Start by looking along the nasal septum. Move your focus to the floor of the nose. Move your focus to the lateral wall of the nose where you should see the inferior turbinate. Move your focus to the upper portion of the nasal cavity where in some noses you may be able to glimpse the middle turbinate and then return to the nasal septum.

Are secretions/discharges present? If so, is the secretion/discharge any of the following?

- Watery – consider CSF rhinorrhoea
- Clear and mucoid – consider viral rhinitis, allergy
- Mucopurulent – consider bacterial rhinitis, sinusitis. (Note: If unilateral, always consider an FB in a child, a tumour in an adult)

- Blood-stained – consider infection, causes for epistaxis, tumour

Is the mucosa any of the following?
- Normal in colour, not too wet, and not too 'thickened' – normal
- Pale, wet, and thickened – consider allergy
- Inflamed, wet, and thickened – consider rhinitis, overuse of decongestant sprays/drops (known as rhinitis medicamentosa)
- 'Cyanosed', not too wet and thickened – consider 'vasomotor rhinitis' (non-allergic rhinitis)

Is the septum any of the following?
- Straight – normal
- Deviated:
  - C-shaped
  - S-shaped
  - spurs
  - other

(If it is deviated, you should consider whether or not the deviation corresponds to symptoms of nasal obstruction.)

Are the blood vessels on the septum particularly prominent?
- Does this correspond with a history of epistaxis?
- Does touching these vessels make them bleed?

Consider cautery.

Are the inferior turbinates any of the following?:
- Symmetrical – normal
- Enlarged – consider rhinitis, allergy, vasomotor rhinitis
- Abnormally small – consider turbinectomy surgery, atrophic rhinitis

Are there any abnormal masses in the nasal cavities?
- FB
- Nasal polyp
- Tumour

If after completing your examination you are unable to determine a cause for the patient's complaint, you will have to consider other likely causes for the complaint that may indicate that the problem area is beyond the limit of your examination, for example adenoid hypertrophy in a child, some form of mass – benign or malignant – in an adult, or a posterior site for epistaxis. Consideration may have to be given to further examination by radiology or to referral for an ENT specialist opinion.

8 Core knowledge of nose and sinus disorders

Vestibulitis and impetigo

The openings to the nasal cavities (the nostrils or nasal vestibules) are lined by hair-bearing skin. This area is subject to trauma, predominantly digital. Any breech of the skin surface predisposes to infection – particularly when associated with a rhinitis. This infection may be localized as a furuncle in a hair follicle or there may be ulceration. If the infection is staphylococcal, it may spread to the surrounding facial skin (impetigo). In addition to these factors, this is a common site for herpes simplex 'cold' sores. Warts are not uncommon. Suspect malignancy in persistent ulceration in adults. Consider use of an antibiotic for any significant infection in this area as it is part of the 'danger area' for infection – some of the venous drainage is backwards and intracranially with potential for an infected cavernous sinus thrombosis. Penicillin (erythromycin) is required for impetigo and a furuncle but usually all that is needed for ulceration is cleansing and application of an antiseptic. A proprietary remedy is useful for cold sores.

Rhinitis/Sinusitis

Rhinitis

Almost everyone will experience episodes of viral rhinitis – the common cold. Apart from systemic malaise making them feel miserable, the nasal mucosa responds with inflammatory swelling (nasal obstruction), irritation (sneezing), and excessive mucus production with impaired ciliary function (rhinorrhoea). The swollen mucosa and impaired ciliary function predisposes to obstruction of the drainage passages (ostia) of the sinuses with accumulation of exudate in the sinuses (feeling of stuffiness in the head and loss of vocal resonance). Treatment of viral rhinitis is not strictly required. Isolation to prevent spread of infection is desirable but not usually practical. Analgesics may ease the viral malaise and steam inhalations may be soothing to the nose, but many patients resort to use of nasal decongestants. The immune system should resolve the infection in a few days. Secondary bacterial infection is common, manifesting by change to a mucopurulent nasal discharge. At this stage infection may spread to the sinuses, the middle ear, the tonsils and adenoid, and the lower respiratory tract. Some patients appear to be predisposed to involvement of one or more of these sites. This secondary bacterial infection may require the use of antibiotics.

Remember to consider syphilis in babies with 'snuffles' – persistent rhinitis.

Remember to consider a foreign body in all cases of unilateral rhinitis in children (often foul-smelling) and tumour in all cases of unilateral rhinitis in adults.

Sinusitis

Sinusitis is usually precipitated by a viral rhinitis and in children the ethmoidal sinuses are as likely to be involved as the maxillary sinus. Dental roots project into the floor of the maxillary sinus and these can be a source of infection. Acute pressure changes, for example during diving, can force contaminated material into the maxillary sinus. The frontal and sphenoidal sinuses only begin to become well pneumatized after about ten years of age, and of these two, the frontal sinus is the more likely to become infected, sphenoidal sinusitis being uncommon (deep-seated headache). The potential to develop sinusitis is exacerbated when the complex drainage channels of the sinuses are obstructed (anatomical abnormalities, oedematous mucosa) or when there is impaired ciliary function. The predominant symptom of sinusitis is pain associated with 'stuffiness' and a mucopurulent nasal discharge. Treatment involves the use of antibiotics and topical nasal decongestants, and should be continued for at least two weeks.

Potential complications. With ethmoidal and frontal sinusitis, infection may spread into the orbit (orbital cellulitis) or into the anterior cranial fossa. Rarely, involvement of venous channels may precipitate a cavernous sinus thrombosis. All such complications require emergency referral to a specialist service.

Inadequate treatment of acute sinusitis predisposes to establishment of chronic sinusitis (nasal obstruction, stuffiness, mucopurulent nasal discharge, or postnasal drip). This predisposition may relate to underlying allergic rhinitis, anatomical deformities in drainage passages or, rarely, cystic fibrosis or mucociliary transport disorders. Failure of resolution after a prolonged course of antibiotic (based on bacterial culture) and nasal decongestant requires referral to a specialist service, since by this stage surgery is probably required.

Atrophic rhinitis

The cause is usually obscure in this, fortunately rare, condition. Atrophy of the nasal mucosa results in excessive drying and crusting of nasal secretions with infection and ulceration of mucosa beneath the crusts further damaging the mucosa. A foul nasal odour is the basis for its other name of ozaena. If cleaning by irrigation and moistening by use of glucose/glycerine drops is not helpful, there are a number of surgical procedures to reduce nasal airflow that may need to be considered.

Allergic rhinitis

Sensitized individuals undergo a Type I hypersensitivity reaction in the nasal mucosa. The allergen binds to IGE on the surface of mast cells within the mucosa, causing mast cell degranulation and the release of two kinds of allergic mediators. Early mediators such as histamine cause vascular dilatation and mucosal oedema (nasal obstruction), mucosal irritation (sneezing), and mucus hypersecretion (rhinorrhoea). Reflex stimulation of parasympathetic nerves perpetuates the nasal congestion. Late mediators promote migration of eosinophils into the mucosa and these release substances such a leukotrienes which are responsible for the persistent nasal congestion. See Table 8.1.

Table 8.1 Allergic rhinitis

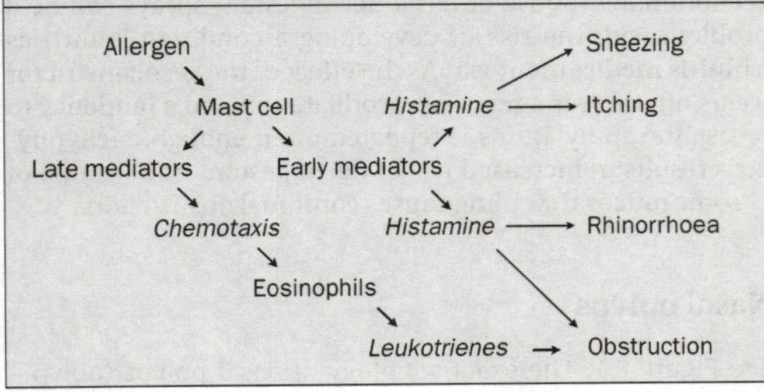

Two broad types of allergic rhinitis are recognized although they are not mutually exclusive – seasonal allergic rhinitis (predominantly pollen) and perennial allergic rhinitis (predominantly house-dust mite and animal dander). A good history usefully serves to distinguish these types. Further investigation by skin prick testing or allergy assay (phadiotype, RAST) may be utilized to identify the specific allergens.

Treatment is by avoidance (usually impractical), antihistamine (useful for acute reactions), 'mast cell stabilizers', such as sodium cromoglycate (useful for seasonal rhinitis), or topical steroid nasal sprays (the mainstay of therapy). Systemic steroids are useful to ameliorate symptoms for important events (exams, interviews, weddings, etc.).

Allergic rhinitis predisposes to acute and chronic sinusitis.

Non-allergic rhinitis

The nasal mucosa of sensitized individuals reacts adversely to irritants – dust, fumes, vapours, pollutants – with similar symptoms to those of allergic rhinitis but with different emphasis – usually a 'dry' nasal obstruction (the term 'vasomotor rhinitis' is often applied to these individuals on the assumption that parasympathetic overactivity is the underlying cause). There is no IGE elevation and specific allergens cannot be identified in these individuals. Hence treatment is often difficult but many respond favourably to topical steroid nasal sprays. In those individuals in whom nasal congestion predominates, abuse of nasal decongestant sprays can be a problem with the risk of developing a condition known as '**rhinitis medicamentosa**'. As the effect of the vasoconstrictor wears off, there is a reactive vasodilatation and a tendency to re-use the spray. If this is repeated often enough, tachyphylaxis results in increased use of decongestant until a state of chronic mucosal swelling causes continual obstruction.

Nasal polyps

See Figure 8.1. The exact aetiology of nasal polyps (polyp – protruding growth from a mucous membrane) is unknown. Simplistically, they arise from the small ethmoidal sinuses when an oedematous reaction in the sinus mucosa causes it to fill the sinus and then protrude through the sinus opening (ostium) to expand within the nasal cavity. Hence they are often associated with nasal allergy and/or asthma. Another frequent association for some unknown reason is with aspirin sensitivity. They are most often bilateral. (Note: Unilateral nasal polyps should always arouse suspicion of neoplasia.) Polyps usually have the appearance of greyish, smooth-surfaced masses but with exposure to the drying effect of air they sometimes acquire a 'mucosal' appearance and the polyp then needs to be distinguished from a turbinate by its insensitivity and mobility when palpated with a probe. The symptoms they produce are of nasal obstruction and, because this extends to obstruction of air flow to the olfactory area in the roof of the nose, loss of the sense of the smell (anosmia).

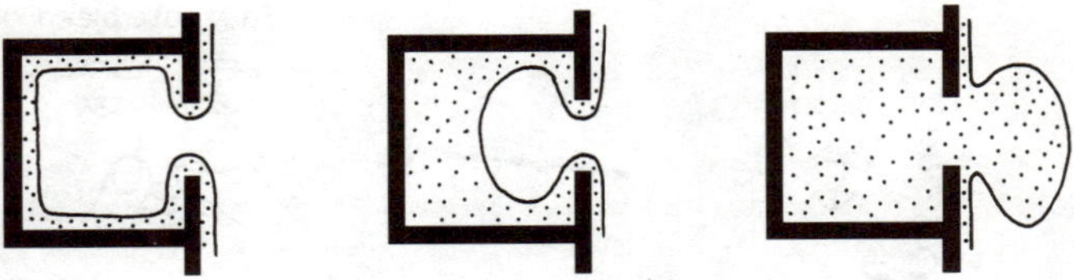

Figure 8.1 Formation of a nasal polyp

Treatment. Polyps may regress after a course of systemic steroid reinforced by topical steroid nasal spray. Failure to respond requires surgical removal followed by topical steroid nasal spray to prevent recurrence. Further recurrence is an indication for sinus surgery.

Epistaxis

Bleeding from the nose is a common problem. Both rhinitis and periods of hot weather seem to predispose to nose bleeds but fortunately 90 per cent of these will arise from the anterior, visible portion of the nasal cavity. These are best thought of as the 'easy' epistaxis because the site of bleeding is frequently from Little's area on the nasal septum. Here it can be controlled by pinching this portion of the nose for a few minutes and this area is also accessible for cautery.

Bleeding from the posterior regions of the nasal cavity tends to present problems in management – the 'difficult' epistaxis. These will usually be adult patients – posterior bleeding is unusual in children – and it is exacerbated when there is co-existing arteriosclerosis and hypertension. Pressure can only be applied in this area by some form of nasal packing and it is sometimes difficult to achieve adequate haemostasis. Examination under anaesthetic and attempts at cautery may be required. As a last resort, ligation of nasal feeding vessels – ethmoidal and maxillary arteries – may be needed. (See Figure 8.2.)

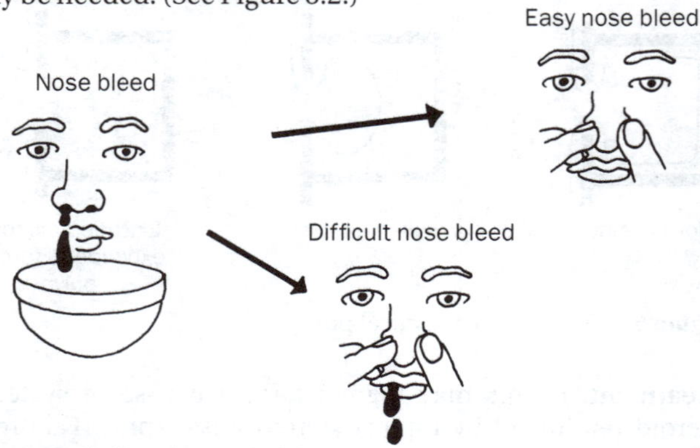

Figure 8.2 Epistaxis

Although most nose bleeds are minor and inconsequential, it has to be remembered that some nose bleeds, particularly posteriorly, can be torrential and life-threatening in themselves and also that they may be an indication of life-threatening disorders – local: nasal tumours; general: blood disorders – anti-coagulants, liver problems, leukaemia, etc.

The list of potential causes for epistaxis includes:

Anterior:
- Rhinitis
- Minor and digital trauma
- Foreign body
- 'Bleeding septal polypus'

Superior:
- Trauma to nasal skeleton

Posterior:
- Spontaneous
- Rhinosinusitis

- Bleeding disorders, anticoagulants, chronic liver disease, blood dyscrasias
- Nasal tumours, particularly the angiofibroma of adolescent males

Generalized:
- Bleeding disorders
- Haemorrhagic telangiectasia (Osler's disease), fortunately rare

Management of epistaxis is detailed in Chapter 9, pp. 120–123.

Nasal septal deviation

Nasal septal deviation is a common finding. It arises either because the septum, during growth, has exceeded the dimensions allowed for it in the nasal cavity (in order to 'fit' it has had to either buckle into a C- or S-shape, or dislocate from its inferior attachment to the floor of the nose), following trauma (this trauma may have occurred during birth when the nose is compressed during passage through the birth canal) or because a mass in one nasal cavity is forcing the septum across the midline into the other side. Septal deviation may cause symptoms of nasal obstruction by its anatomical shape which alters the normal pattern of air flow but more usually the turbinates expand to fill any extra capacity created in the nasal cavity by the septal deformity. The indications for surgery are either nasal obstruction or cosmetic deformity of the cartilaginous nasal skeleton. Surgery involves reducing the septal cartilage dimensions, straightening cartilage angulation, and removing areas of bony septal deformity. See Figure 8.3. Care has to be taken to assess the extent of turbinate hypertrophy and to reduce turbinate bulk when required. Potential complications of surgery are loss of septal cartilage with consequent 'saddle' deformity of the cartilaginous nasal skeleton and septal perforation.

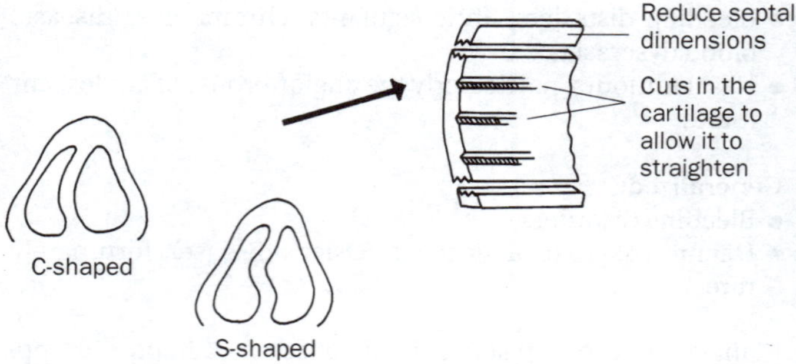

Figure 8.3 Septoplasty

Nasal trauma

Blunt trauma to the nose is a common problem. The mechanism of injury is divided into lateral injuries (lateral displacement) and frontal injuries (depression). See Figure 8.4. Bony components of the nasal skeleton tend to fracture, cartilage components tend to buckle (but may also fracture). In the assessment of nasal trauma, two questions have to be answered. The first is 'Has the patient broken his nose?' (local tenderness and swelling). The second is 'Is the skeleton displaced?' (visible deformity, obstructed airway). Displacement is the indication for manipulation.

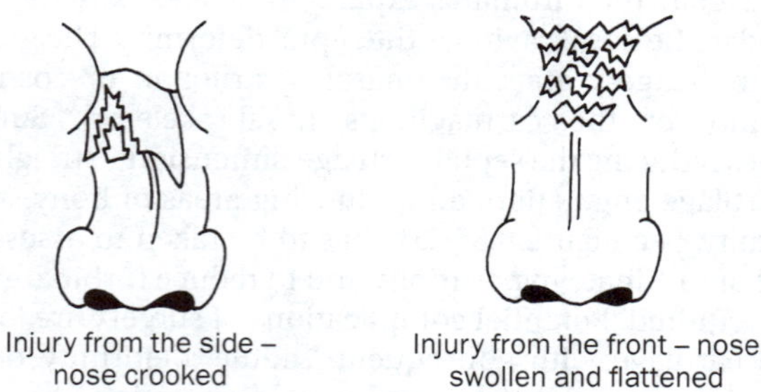

Figure 8.4 Nasal trauma

Manipulation is usually undertaken a week to ten days after injury when swelling will have settled enough to assess the extent of displacement and the results of manipulation. However, there are potential complications from septal injury which require urgent referral. See Figure 8.5. When a haematoma forms beneath the septal mucosa it tends to become rapidly infected and the resulting septal abscess invariably destroys the septal cartilage with an end result of a depressed 'saddle' nasal profile. Urgent drainage and antibiotics may salvage the septal cartilage.

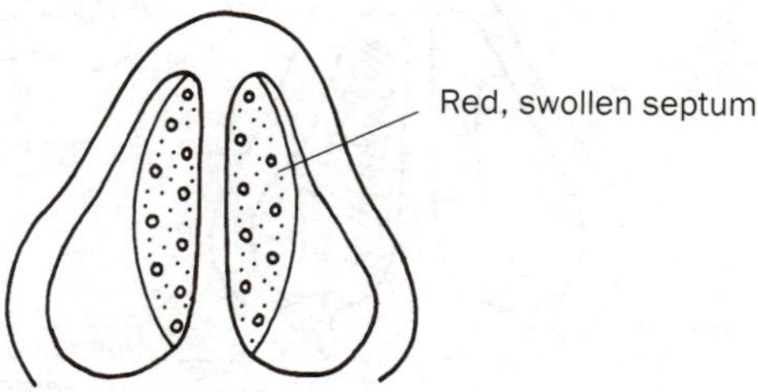

Figure 8.5 Nasal septum haematoma

Septal trauma as a result of repetitive digital trauma, repeated cauterization, or septal surgery may cause a septal perforation.

Paediatric rhinology

Choanal atresia

Choanal atresia (rare, occurring in about 1:20 000 births) is a condition in which the posterior openings of the nasal cavity into the nasopharynx fail to develop. Neonates are obligatory nasal breathers and will not breathe through their mouths if the nasal passages are obstructed unless an airway is strapped in place. This is the emergency treatment for choanal atresia. After confirmation of the diagnosis, either by direct examination with an endoscope or use of contrast radiology, the choanal openings are created surgically.

Foreign bodies

Foreign bodies are a common problem (see Figure 8.6). Small children frequently put objects into their own and other children's body orifices – often the nose. Stasis of secretions around the object predisposes to infection with a foul smell and a mucopurulent, sometimes blood-stained, unilateral nasal discharge. Removal (see *Removal of a foreign body from the nose*, Chapter 14) resolves the situation.

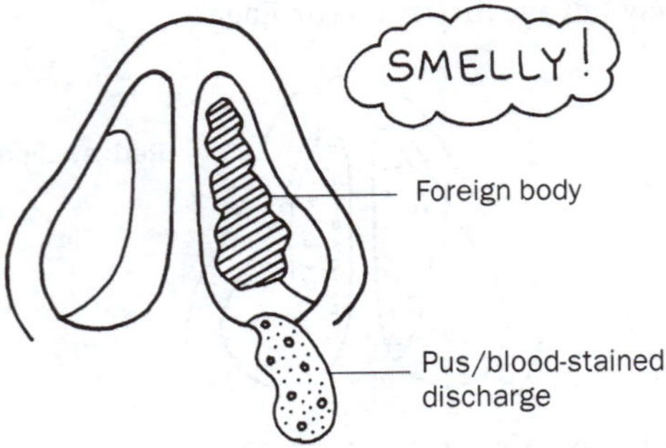

Figure 8.6 Foreign body in the nose

Adenoids

The adenoid is the first site of contact between lymphoid tissue and inhaled allergens, organisms, and pathogens. Hence in infancy it is in a constant state of hyperactivity as the body reacts to develop immunity to all these factors. The most common cause of upper airway obstruction in childhood is adenoid hypertrophy.

Upper airway obstruction itself is common in infants and small children and is always associated with persistent snoring and mouth breathing. The more severe degrees of obstruction are associated with restless, disturbed sleep, enuresis, and struggling for breath when sleeping. At its worst this struggling manifests with episodes of obstructive apnoea (which may be one cause for Sudden Infant Death Syndrome – SIDS). Failure to thrive is frequent in these more severely obstructed infants (a lot of energy is involved in breathing against an obstruction) and prolonged obstruction may precipitate cardiac failure (hypoxia – pulmonary vasoconstriction – pulmonary hypertension – cor pulmonale – cardiac failure).

Adenoiditis is one source for ascending infection of the middle ear via the eustachian tube (acute otitis media) and adenoid hypertrophy is a common cause of eustachian tube dysfunction (middle ear effusions). Check the ears and hearing of snoring infants and children.

These symptoms are all indications for referral to an ENT specialist service for removal of adenoids (adenoidectomy).

Snoring

The negative pressure in the upper airway generated during inspiratory efforts not only causes ingress of air but also inward prolapse of the soft tissue walls and any protruding masses, for example tonsils and tongue (Bernoulli effect). If this prolapse is sufficient to cause air-flow obstruction, the negative pressure increases, the obstruction is overcome, air flow returns, prolapse recurs, and a cycle is established. The vibrations created produce the characteristic sound known as stertor or snoring. See Figure 8.7.

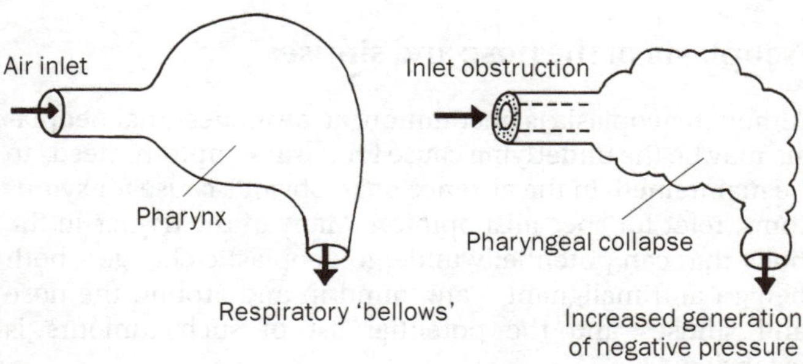

Figure 8.7 Obstruction as a contribution to snoring

Snoring is a common problem both in children (see above) and in adults. Not only is it disruptive to others but it also has serious implications for the snorer (see above, the same mechanism operates in adults). In adults, snoring is predominantly vibratory (for example lax soft palate and uvula), predominantly obstructive (usually associated with obesity), or a combination of both.

The basis of treatment is to identify factors contributing to obstruction of air inflow into the upper airway. Relieve the obstruction and less negative pressure generation is required for air inflow. The nasal airway is the narrowest portion of the airway and factors operating here that contribute to snoring include:

- Excessive narrowing or collapse of the 'nasal valve' area – see Chapter 7, page 97
- Enlarged nasal turbinates
- Deviated nasal septum
- Nasal polyps and other nasal 'masses'
- Adenoids in children, nasopharyngeal tumours in children and adults.

Other factors to be considered are pharyngeal – soft palate/ uvula, tonsils, pharyngeal and parapharyngeal 'masses' – and laryngeal disorders (stridor can be mistaken for stertor).

Treatment is directed to the affected anatomical area and its abnormality.

Neoplasia of the nose and sinuses

Although neoplasia is uncommon, an awareness that neoplasia may be the underlying cause for nasal symptoms needs to be maintained. In the absence of an obvious cause for symptoms, refer for specialist opinion. Many of the tissues in the body that can potentially undergo neoplastic change – both benign and malignant – are found in and around the nose and sinuses and the potential list of such tumours is extensive.

Dictums to remember are:

- The cause for unilateral nasal obstruction always needs to be determined.
- Unilateral nasal discharge in a child is usually caused by a foreign body but in an adult a tumour needs to be excluded.
- Beware of unilateral middle ear effusion in an adult – a nasopharyngeal tumour always needs to be excluded.
- Beware of a blood-stained nasal discharge – a nasal tumour always needs to be excluded even though the most common cause is infection.
- Beware of the 'node in the neck' with no obvious primary neoplasia. The nasopharynx is one area for a hidden primary.
- Be aware of aetiological factors – smoking, snuff usage, wood-workers (adenocarcinoma).

The general principles of management that apply to neoplasia of the nose and sinuses are similar to those that apply for other ENT areas in which neoplasia occurs. These are given in more detail in Chapter 12, pages 159–160. In summary, these principles include:

- Diagnosis by suspicion, examination, and biopsy
- Assessment and staging – TNM system
- Therapy – modalities include:
  - Surgery – this encompasses ablation, reconstruction, prosthetics, rehabilitation, and support
  - Chemotherapy
  - Radiotherapy
  - Other – for example hormone manipulation for pituitary tumours
- Follow up to detect recurrent disease, second primaries, and distant metastasis
- Terminal care when the disease becomes incurable

9 A practical approach to nose and sinus disorders

As noted previously, most patients do not know exactly what they are suffering from. They usually complain about a collection of symptoms and expect you to tell them what is wrong. Without specialized equipment and skills, examination of the nose will reveal only cosmetic deformities and anteriorly situated pathology or deformity. Therefore a practical approach is largely based on patient symptoms. The symptoms arising from nasal and sinus disorders are described below.

Symptoms

- Nasal obstruction
- Nasal discharge (rhinorrhoea) and postnasal drip
- Pain
- Epistaxis (bleeding)
- Sneezing
- Snoring
- Loss of vocal resonance
- Loss of smell
- Cosmetic deformity

Nasal obstruction

The sensation of nasal obstruction is very subjective and it may sometimes be difficult to determine the cause. It is relatively easy when there is an obvious obstructing element but the dimensions of the nasal cavity vary tremendously as the mucosa swells and shrinks not only with the 'nasal cycle' but under the influence of the autonomic system and in response to allergens and irritants. If you add to this the need for rigidity or support of the airway walls, and the effects on these walls of muscle relaxation when sleeping, it can be seen that the situation pertaining at the time of consultation may not be representative of the situation when the sensation of obstruction is at its worst. Another factor that seems to play a role in the sensation of obstruction is alteration of the pattern of air flow through the nasal cavity. Some patients may complain of an obstructive sensation even when the nasal passages appear to be adequate.

Potential causes and treatment

The underlying disorders that may potentially cause nasal obstruction are described below.

Infection, such as viral rhinitis, acute and chronic bacterial rhinosinusitis, is always accompanied by mucosal swelling and nasal discharge. Viral rhinitis should need no more than symptomatic treatment for the malaise but many patients resort to decongestants, either systemic or topical. The onset of facial pain may be indicative of acute sinusitis, usually heralded by a change from mucoid to purulent discharge, and this should be treated with an antibiotic and topical nasal decongestant to improve drainage from the sinuses. Inadequately treated acute sinusitis may progress to chronicity with purulent nasal and postnasal discharge. A deep nasal swab should be taken to guide a much longer course of antibiotic and decongestant.

Allergic rhinitis is suggested when there is a triad of nasal obstruction, watery or mucoid discharge, and sneezing in response to exposure to an allergen. The allergen can usually be identified from a carefully taken history – seasonal is usually due to pollens, perennial is most often due to house-dust mite but may also be caused by moulds and animal dander. Often the patient can identify the allergen when the allergic response is caused by a known contact such as animal dander, or by a situation such as a particular room or building. Antihistamines and sodium cromoglycate are useful for contact or seasonal rhinitis but perennial rhinitis usually requires topical nasal steroids.

Non-allergic rhinitis is in many ways similar to allergic rhinitis but one symptom – usually nasal obstruction – predominates. There is a strong element of parasympathetic overactivity to this disorder – 'My nose always blocks up in a stuffy room', '… in the evening', etc. – and characteristically the inferior turbinates are enlarged with a rather cyanotic appearance. It is a much more difficult disorder to treat – good response to topical decongestants tends to lead patients to overuse these with ensuing problems of rebound congestion and eventual rhinitis medicamentosa, and they should be avoided. Some patients respond well to topical nasal steroids but many require referral for surgery to reduce the bulk of the offending turbinates.

Anatomical deformity – deviated nasal septum, nasal 'valve' collapse – is suspected when nasal obstruction is present all the time. Careful examination should detect the underlying abnormality and when this is a septal deviation the turbinate in the nasal passage with more space is often enlarged – compensatory hypertrophy. These patients require referral for assessment for surgical correction of the deformity.

Nasal polyps are often associated with allergy, although this is more often asthma than allergic rhinitis, and present with nasal obstruction and loss of smell. Polyps can usually be seen in the nose and sometimes have to be distinguished from an enlarged turbinate – a turbinate is sensitive when touched with a probe whereas a polyp is insensitive. They are usually bilateral and treatment is with a short course of systemic steroid supplemented by topical nasal steroids which are continued for three months. This should shrink most polyps but if they do not respond or recur, referral for nasal polypectomy will be required. There is a variant – the antrochoanal polyp – that arises on one side only and is unresponsive to steroids. It can grow to such a size that it protrudes either anteriorly or posteriorly from the nasal cavity.

Adenoid hypertrophy is the most common cause of nasal obstruction and snoring in children. There is not a lot that can be done to shrink the adenoid but any nasal allergy or rhinitis should be treated. The indications for referral for adenoidectomy include persistent nasal obstruction, snoring associated with airway obstruction when sleeping, recurrent middle ear infection, and persistent middle ear effusions.

Nasal and nasopharyngeal tumours should be suspected when there is a history of recent onset of nasal obstruction. The other sinister sign associated with a tumour is bleeding or a blood-stained nasal discharge. Sometimes the presence of a malignant tumour may produce no symptoms until a neck node appears. Any suspicion of a tumour is an indication for an urgent referral.

Rhinorrhoea (nasal discharge) and postnasal drip

Up to 750 ml of watery mucus can be produced daily by the nasal mucosa to assist its air-conditioning function. Normally this is propelled posteriorly by the mucosal cilia. Any increase in production may be perceived as 'catarrh' or 'postnasal drip'. Posterior obstruction (for example adenoids in children) may cause stasis and accumulation of secretions.

When the normal situation is altered and there is a nasal discharge, the character of the discharge is perhaps the most helpful factor in determining the aetiology of any underlying disorder.

Potential causes and treatment

Watery/mucoid:
- Viral rhinitis
- Allergic rhinitis

These have been discussed in the previous section on nasal obstruction.
- CSF leaks are very uncommon. They are usually precipitated by trauma that is associated with a fracture of the cribriform plate but on rare occasions may be congenital when they are associated with recurrent meningitis. CSF is distinguished from other watery nasal discharges by the presence of glucose and this is easily tested by using a glucose 'dipstick'.

Mucopurulent:
- Bacterial infective rhinitis
- Acute and chronic sinusitis
- Nasal polyps
These have been discussed in the previous section on nasal obstruction.
- Unilateral purulent discharges should raise suspicion of a FB in children or a tumour in adults. In children the discharge is often associated with a foul smell. Children usually need to be restrained to examine the nose, which can often be done by tilting up the tip of the nose with a finger. Any discharge needs to be sucked away to see what is behind it. To see further back into the nose try using an otoscope. If a FB is seen, try removing it – see Chapter 14, page 193.

Blood-stained:
- Epistaxis is considered in a separate section later in this chapter.
- Infection. Most blood-stained nasal discharges are associated with infection but this diagnosis should be made only after excluding all other causes.
- Trauma. CSF leaks associated with trauma were mentioned above. Initially these are blood-stained. Digital trauma is very common and children have a habit of putting a variety of other things up their noses that can precipitate minor bleeds and blood-staining of nasal discharges. Trauma also includes things like vigorous nose blowing which, particularly when there is nasal infection, may precipitate a small bleed.

- Neoplasia. Blood-stained, unilateral nasal discharges are always indicative of tumours and if there is nothing obvious to see when examining the nose an urgent referral is necessary.

Pain

Pain arising from nasal and sinus disorders usually remains localized in this anatomical area although there may not be precision in localization. Potential disorders that may cause pain are described below.

Potential causes and treatment

Vestibulitis/vestibular furuncle. These should be obvious on examination. Vestibulitis is often due to herpetic infection and needs no more than application of a proprietary cold sore remedy. When there is added bacterial infection, children often disseminate this by scratching until it becomes a frank impetigo. Antiseptic cream and a systemic antibiotic should clear this. An antibiotic should be considered for furuncles as this is the 'danger area' of the face with venous drainage backwards into the cavernous sinus.

Acute and chronic sinusitis. Acute sinusitis is always painful but when sinusitis becomes chronic, pain has more the character of discomfort or headaches associated with nasal stuffiness. Some clues as to which sinus is involved are obtained from the distribution of the pain:

- Maxillary – in the cheek or upper dentition
- Ethmoidal – between the eyes
- Frontal – above the eyes, tends to be exacerbated by bending over
- Sphenoidal – deep-seated

It is reasonable to treat acute sinusitis on clinical diagnosis from a history of a recent cold, onset of pain and purulent nasal discharge, and both an antibiotic and topical nasal decongestants should be given. Chronic sinusitis requires X-rays for a definitive diagnosis and the treatment is initially with a two to three week course of antibiotic – best guided by a deep nasal swab – and topical nasal decongestants to improve drainage. Failure to clear the infection is an indication to refer for some sort of sinus drainage procedure.

Neuralgia from pressure on the middle turbinate by a deviated septum. This may be the cause of troublesome, recurrent, deeper seated pain. It is not an easy diagnosis to make, since often this area of the nasal cavity cannot be easily seen. Such patients should be referred for more detailed examination. Once diagnosed, the treatment is to straighten the nasal septum and relieve the pressure. Pain in and around the eyes may be a part of other neuralgias and migraine headaches that have facial pain as part of the symptomatology.

Neoplasia is an ever-present worry when there is persistent pain in and around the nose and, if there is nothing to find on examination, can only be excluded by both specialist examination and radiology.

Epistaxis (bleeding)

Patients may present either actively bleeding or with a history of epistaxis.

Active bleeding. These patients will initially require first aid measures to control the bleeding. These follow a stepwise progression:

- Ninety per cent of epistaxis arises anteriorly in the nose (the 'easy' epistaxis) and this can usually be controlled by requesting the patient to sit upright, lean forward, and pinch the nose. The effect of pressure can be enhanced with some vasoconstriction – soak a piece of cotton wool in adrenaline or one of the nasal vasoconstrictor drops, place this in the nose, and apply pressure.
- For the remainder with posterior bleeding (the 'difficult' epistaxis) – these will almost always be adults since posterior bleeding is uncommon in children – pinching the nose will result in the blood trickling posteriorly into the

pharynx. To apply pressure posteriorly implies some form of packing (see Figure 9.1) and this is so unpleasant for the patient that it is worth trying to spray vasoconstrictor deep into the nasal cavity and waiting a few minutes to see whether the bleeding will stop before resorting to packing. If it doesn't, the nasal cavity will have to be packed deeply. Many of these patients with posterior bleeds are middle-aged or elderly and absorption of vasoconstrictors, particularly adrenaline, will have cardiac side-effects. Therefore use either Vaseline® gauze or ribbon gauze soaked in BIPP.

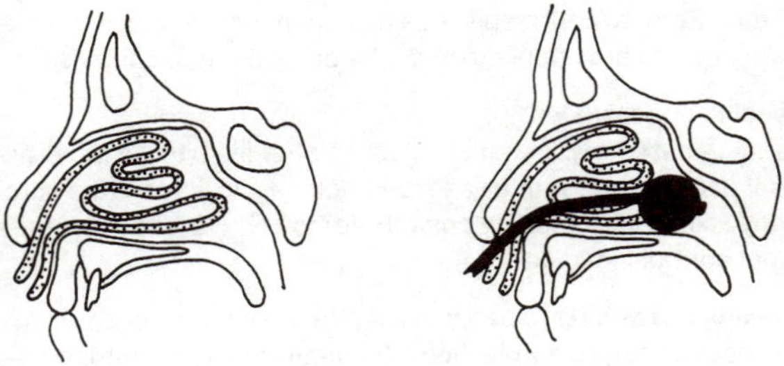

Figure 9.1 Control of epistaxis

- If there is still a significant amount of blood trickling posteriorly after packing, some form of tamponade of the posterior choana will be required. (See Figure 9.1.) The most useful method is to pass a Foley catheter through the nasal cavity, inject 5 ml of water into the bulb, and draw the catheter forwards until the bulb impacts in the choana. If the nasal packing had to be removed to do this it will need to be replaced.
- R All of these patients with posterior bleeds require referral for admission to an ENT specialist service. So once the bleeding is controlled, check for signs of hypovolaemic shock, set up an intravenous fluid line, resuscitate if necessary, take blood for cross-matching if there has been significant blood loss, check for systemic causes – anticoagulants, liver dysfunction, blood dyscrasias – then treat

appropriately and arrange for transfer. If this will be delayed admit locally for strict bed rest with sedation and half-hourly pulse and blood pressure monitoring. See Table 9.1 below.

Table 9.1 Epistaxis

Bleeding: Pinch nose

Bleeding controlled:
Examine the nose for pathology or for a bleeding point requiring cautery. Refer to ENT if epistaxis has been recurrent and troublesome and you are unable to find a bleeding point to cauterize.

Bleeding uncontrolled:
Bleeding anteriorly. Try pinching again after inserting a superficial nasal pack soaked with a vasoconstrictor. Follow this with cautery of any accessible bleeding point. Refer to ENT if these measures do not control bleeding.

Bleeding posteriorly (blood trickles into the pharynx even when the nose is adequately pinched.) Try instilling vasoconstrictor as drops/spray or soaked into a deep nasal pack. If bleeding remains uncontrolled, insert a postnasal balloon and repack. All these patients need to be admitted for bed rest and sedation or to be referred for ENT admission.

Not actively bleeding. Obtain a good history and then examine the nose to see if an identifiable cause or accessible bleeding site can be identified.

- Consider removal of the cause (digital trauma, foreign body) or treatment of the cause (infection, bleeding disorder).
- Consider cautery of the bleeding point (see *Cauterizing the nose*, Chapter 14) if the bleeding has been recurrent or the vessel is particularly prominent.
- (R) Consider referral for specialist management if there is:
  - anterior or posterior bleeding uncontrolled by first aid measures (resuscitation, bed rest, and sedation while awaiting referral).

- posterior bleeding that has required packing/tamponade for control (resuscitation, bed rest, and sedation while awaiting referral).
- an identified cause requiring specialist management (nasal skeletal trauma, bleeding polyp, nasal tumour, haemorrhagic telangiectasia, bleeding disorders).
- troublesome bleeding for which a cause or a site have not been identified.

Sneezing

A cause for sporadic sneezing can usually be identified – a list of potential causes is given below – and removal of the cause or treatment/resolution of the disorder may resolve the problem. Patients often need a little prompting to help them identify precipitating factors or situations which they may then be able to avoid. Disabling, persistent, uncontrollable sneezing (fortunately rare) usually has no identifiable cause but may result from brain-stem pathology.

Potential causes

- Infection – particularly viral rhinitis
- Irritants
- Allergic rhinitis
- Non-allergic rhinitis, especially with temperature change and bright light
- Foreign body

Snoring

Potential causes

Snoring or stertor is the sound produced by vibrating tissue in the upper airway. Simple vibratory snoring is produced by turbulent air flow. However, there is a more sinister aspect to snoring since it usually indicates a greater or lesser degree of airway obstruction (see Chapter 8, page 111), a situation with potential complications. In children with this type of obstructive snoring the usual cause will be enlarged adenoids. In adults it is most commonly associated with obesity.

Treatment

In a practical approach to snoring the history is of prime importance in determining the need for intervention but unfortunately the patient is unable to provide the relevant history, apart from the effects of the resulting disturbed sleep. The observations of those others affected by the snoring are needed for this information but are not always available. In this situation one often has to resort to admission and observation – at its most sophisticated in a 'sleep laboratory'. Apart from the usual information regarding onset, duration, etc. one needs to know about the degree of obstruction associated with the snoring. Does the patient appear to struggle for breath? Is there sternal recession or rib retraction? Are there episodes of obstructive apnoea? Does the patient become cyanosed?

Examination is of importance in directing intervention. There are two elements to this. First, identify vibrating structures in the pharynx, which is usually a lax soft palate with an enlarged uvula. Second, identify anything obstructing inspiratory air inflow that causes an increase in the negative pressure generated by inspiratory efforts that in turn causes soft tissue structures in the upper airway to prolapse, exacerbating the situation. These latter include:

- 'Nasal valve' collapse
- Deviation of nasal septum
- Turbinate hypertrophy
- Nasal polyps, nasal tumours
- Adenoids in children
- Nasopharyngeal tumours in adults – lymphoma, carcinoma
- Enlarged tonsils

- Retropharyngeal and parapharyngeal 'masses' – abscess, nodes, tumours

Having obtained an overall picture of the problem and identified potential causes, appropriate referral can be made. Management relates to both of the above elements. As a first step, any cause for inspiratory air-flow obstruction should be treated or surgically removed. Then vibrating structures should be considered for procedures to reduce bulk or 'tighten up' laxity, for example uvulo-palato-pharyngoplasty.

Loss of vocal resonance

Three mechanisms operate in altering the resonant quality of the voice. 'Nasal escape' imparts a quality known as hypernasality and nasal obstruction a quality known as hyponasality. The main causes for these are listed below. A mass in the pharynx imparts a quality known as a 'hot potato' voice.

Potential causes and treatment

Hypernasality:
- Palatal defects, particularly cleft palate
- Palatal paralysis – diphtheria in children, bulbar and pseudobulbar palsy
- Destructive disease or surgery

Some form of reconstructive surgery may be possible in some of these patients but by and large the results of surgery are not very satisfactory in improving the vocal quality.

Hyponasality:
- Rhinosinusitis
- Allergic rhinitis
- Non-allergic rhinitis
- Nasal polyps

- Adenoids in children
- Nasal and nasopharyngeal tumours in adults

Vocal quality generally improves with treatment of these disorders but conditions such as allergic rhinitis and nasal polyps tend to be chronic or recurrent and anatomical defects may be the end result of treatment of tumours.

'Hot potato' voice:
- Pharyngeal tumours
- Inflammatory swellings and masses in the pharynx

The change in voice is only part of the problem in these conditions and airway obstruction is more usually the prime consideration.

Loss of smell

Taste and smell are intimately linked and it as well to be aware that many patients may not clearly distinguish between these when trying to describe their symptoms.

Potential causes and treatment

In a similar manner to hearing loss, loss of smell may be considered as either conductive or sensorineural. A list of potential causes is given below.

Conductive causes:
- Viral rhinitis
- Allergic rhinitis
- Acute and chronic sinusitis
- Nasal polyps
- Tumours

The sense of smell should return when these conditions are treated but it has to be remembered that conditions such as allergic rhinitis and nasal polyps tend to be chronic or recurrent. Treatment of tumours may leave anatomical defects and radiotherapy is permanently damaging to the sensory mucosa.

Sensorineural:
- Viral olfactory neuritis
- Trauma to cribriform plate
- Neurosurgical procedures in the anterior cranial fossa

It is unusual to regain the sense of smell after these disorders.

Cosmetic deformity

Potential causes and treatment

The nose occupies a very prominent position on the face and consequently tends to be a focus for attention. Body image is a very personal concept and tolerance of any deformity perceived or obvious varies tremendously. This is entering the realm of cosmetic rhinoplasty surgery which at its most refined can sculpt a nose into a desired shape but is more often used to improve the grosser deformities. There is another element to nasal deformities that has to be taken into consideration in determining the need for corrective surgery, which is more the concern of ENT. It is the extent to which the deformity is causing nasal airway obstruction, since it is important to relieve obstruction when undertaking any corrective procedure on the deformity.

The list of causes for the grosser nasal cosmetic deformities includes:
- **Congenital** – particularly cleft lips and palates.
- **Growth** – humps, septal deviation, tip deformities.
- **Ageing** – drooping tip, rhinophyma (hypertrophy of sebaceous glands over the nasal tip).
- **Trauma** – lateral trauma causes deviation, frontal trauma causes depression. These injuries may be associated with lacerations and scarring. Septal surgery can result in a 'saddle' depression if there is loss of cartilage support.

- Gross **nasal polyposis** and **nasal tumours** cause expansion of the nasal skeleton.
- **Infection** – both septal abscess with loss of cartilage and tertiary syphilis with bone destruction cause 'saddle' depressions. TB causes fibrosis and contracture in the vestibular area. 'Noma' or 'cancrum oris' result in loss of tissue and gross deformity.

PART III
The throat, head, and neck

10 Structure and function of the throat, head, and neck

The head and neck region is one of the most complicated anatomical regions. A sound knowledge of the anatomy is an essential prerequisite before embarking on any surgery of this area, but it is beyond the scope of this textbook. This chapter will focus on those clinically significant structures within the upper aerodigestive tract required for primary ENT care.

The oral cavity

The mucosal lining of the anatomically complex oral cavity is the site of most oral cavity diseases but within the cavity are three clinically significant structures: the dentition, the salivary gland openings, and the tongue.

The dentition

There are four jaw quadrants, sensibly labelled 1, 2, 3, and 4. As you face the patient and move clockwise: 1 is the patient's upper right (if you are on top and right you are no. 1), 2 is upper left, 3 is lower left, and 4 is lower right. There are 32 teeth in the adult jaw, 8 in each quadrant labelled (from the midline) 1, 2, 3, 4, 5, 6, 7, and 8 (central incisor, lateral incisor, canine, 1st premolar, 2nd premolar, 1st molar, 2nd molar, 3rd molar or wisdom). A binary code immediately identifies the tooth you are concerned with, 11 (not eleven but one-one) is the upper right central incisor, and 38 (three-eight) the lower left wisdom. Deciduous teeth are 20 in number, 5 per quadrant, and labelled from the midline a, b, c, d, e.

The salivary gland openings

Stensen's ducts from the parotid glands open on the inner surface of the cheek adjacent to the 2nd upper molar teeth. Wharton's ducts from the submandibular glands open in the floor of the mouth on either side of the frenulum of the tongue. The sublingual glands have multiple ducts that either open into Wharton's duct or independently into the floor of the mouth where they are not obvious. The autonomic innervation to the parotid gland – predominantly serous secretion – is via the otic ganglion which receives its fibres by way of the tympanic plexus located on the medial wall of the middle ear. That of the submandibular gland – a mixture of serous and mucoid saliva – is the submandibular ganglion which receives its fibres by way of the chorda tympani nerve which runs across the middle ear. This arrangement means that these nerves are accessible should denervation of these glands be contemplated, for example to control drooling. Saliva predominantly lubricates food to facilitate mastication and deglutition, but is also essential for oral hygiene (it contains IgA which has a protective role), for taste, and it contains digestive enzymes. A moist environment is also needed for articulation.

The tongue

This muscular (motor innervation is the hypoglossal nerve) and mobile structure is obvious and familiar but remember that the anterior two-thirds, covered by cornified squamous epithelium and the filiform papillae, is touchable, trigeminal tongue but the posterior one-third, behind the circumvallate papillae, is untouchable, glossopharyngeal tongue (gag reflex – be careful how far you put in a tongue depressor). There are numerous taste buds, posteriorly innervated by the glossopharyngeal nerve but anteriorly having afferent fibres that travel via the lingual and chorda tympani nerves (the latter traverses the middle ear where it can be damaged during middle ear surgery). Tasting of food is highly complex. Only the primary tastes of salt, sweet, sour, and bitter are perceived by the tongue, nuances of flavour are olfactory (you can't taste your food with a heavy cold). The piquancy of chilli is 5th nerve with a perverted excitation of sensory fibres.

The mouth and oral cavity are predominantly concerned with grinding up food by the teeth, mixture with liquid saliva, exposure to the digestive enzymes, and backward displacement of the bolus into the oropharynx – the voluntary, first phase of swallowing. Other functions include tasting of food, surveillance of the immunological scene, and forming words.

The pharynx

The entrance to the oropharynx (see Figure 10.1) is framed by the tongue inferiorly, the uvula and soft palate superiorly and, on either side, by the tonsils enclosed fore and aft in a muscular sling, the anterior and posterior faucial pillars. Because the pillars comprise muscle covered by mucosa they are generally red (aemic) – this is often misinterpreted as hyperaemia.

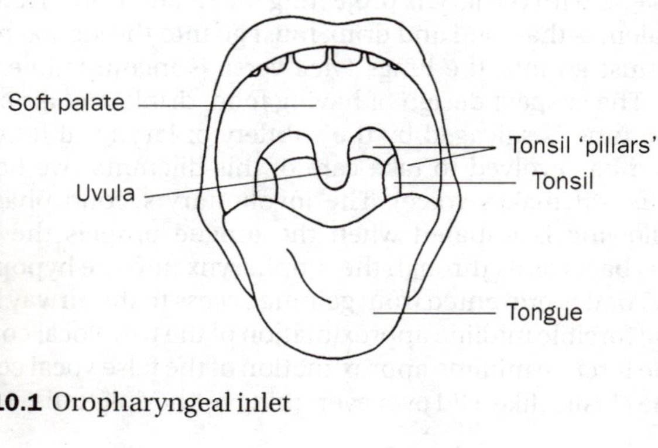

Fig. 10.1 Oropharyngeal inlet

Lymphoid tissue

There is a whole ring of lymphoid tissue (Waldeyer's ring) surrounding and immunologically surveying the upper aerodigestive tract. The largest aggregations are found in the tonsils and the adenoid (situated in the nasopharynx). There is a further aggregation in the base of the tongue (lingual tonsil) and a scattering of small nodules on the posterior pharyngeal wall and behind the posterior faucial pillar. Unlike other lymph glands, these have no afferents, only efferents. Afferent supply is from the surface, with air and food particles passing over the irregular surfaces and becoming trapped. Exposure of B and T lymphocytes to antigenic particles is the first step to full immunologic competence. Not surprisingly, Waldeyer's ring is at its most active in the first few years of life when 'tonsillitis' may be almost thought of as physiological rather than pathological.

The oropharynx

The oropharynx is an ill-defined area between the nasopharynx above and the hypopharynx below.

The hypopharynx

The hypopharynx is the area of the parting of the air and food passages with the larynx projecting into it anteriorly. Here the problem is that food and drink must go into the stomach and air must go into the lungs (vice versa is incompatible with life). The suspect design of having food, drink, and air in the same tube is salvaged by the subtlety of laryngeal function which has evolved to take care of this dilemma (we have a bonus – it makes voice). The involuntary second phase of swallowing is initiated when the tongue propels the food bolus backwards through the oropharynx into the hypopharynx. Food is prevented from gaining access to the airway by:

- the forcible midline approximation of the true vocal cords.
- the forcible midline approximation of the false vocal cords.
- the closing like a lid over everything by the epiglottis.

With the airway sealed, muscular propulsion will get the food or drink to its correct destination.

Of necessity, with air being sucked in by the negative pressure generated during the inspiratory phase of respiration, the airways are rigid and uncollapsible. If the upper airway did not have a certain rigidity, it would collapse like an uninflated balloon (incompatible with life). The laryngeal skeleton may be felt in the neck – the hyoid above, the thyroid and cricoid cartilages suspended beneath this, and then the tracheal rings. In contrast, the food passage is a floppy distensible muscular tube, relying on gravity and muscular contractions of great co-ordination (swallowing) to convey the food to the GIT – the third phase of swallowing.

The larynx

The larynx as a sphincter

The first line of defence of the airway lies at the true cords. The cricoid cartilage, with its two high posterior shoulders, lies below and partially within the arch of the thyroid cartilage – the inferior cornua articulate with the cricoid and clasp it. On top of the shoulders are situated the arytenoid cartilages, highly mobile from side to side. Attached to each is a membrane running forward to the inner surface of the midpoint of the thyroid cartilage (see Figure 10.2). Thus, if the arytenoid cartilages are together (adducted), the edges of this membrane lie side by side, that is they close. If the arytenoids are distracted (abducted), the posterior end opens out creating a V-shaped aperture (the glottis). These movements result from contractions of the laryngeal muscles innervated by the recurrent laryngeal nerves. The membrane is most confusingly called a vocal cord – it is not a cord at all, it has a free edge medially and extends the whole way laterally to be attached onto the side wall of the laryngeal skeleton.

The epiglottis is a leaf-shaped cartilage, rising out of the larynx from its stalk-like attachment just above where the cords meet on the inner surface of the thyroid cartilage. It is ordinarily held vertically, but if allowed to fall backwards, it

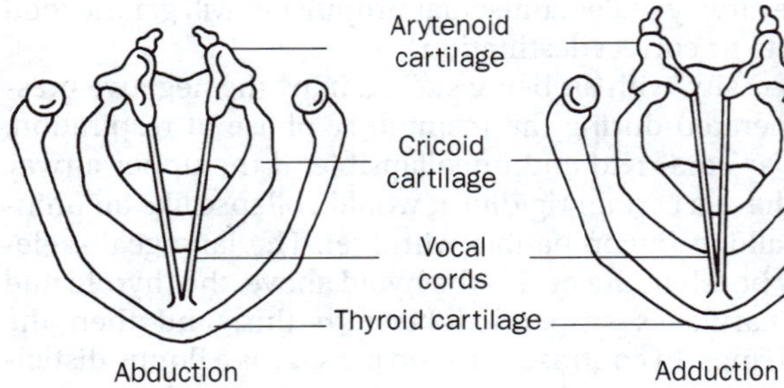

Figure 10.2 Vocal cord movement

closes like a lid over the laryngeal inlet. From both lateral edges of the leaf, swooping down to the arytenoids, are the aryepiglottic folds, which have medial free edges lying above the vocal cords and which are also capable of meeting in the midline. These medial free edges are known as the false cords – the vocal cords are often referred to as true cords.

Thus, the laryngeal phase of swallowing is in three parts, true cord closure, false cord closure, and epiglottic closure, the three together sealing off the airway. With the airway sealed, food and drink are diverted into lateral channels on either side of the epiglottis – the piriform fossae. The opening to the upper oesophagus (the cricopharyngeus muscle sphincter) then relaxes to accommodate the bolus and it is transported by peristaltic muscle contractions to the stomach – the third phase of swallowing.

The larynx as a vocal organ

The physical fact of something vibrating in a column of air is the basis of all wind instruments, including the human voice. The vocal cords are set in motion by the passage of expired air across them (Bernoulli phenomenon) – the basic sound so produced being exemplified by humming. This sound can be modified by doing things with the lips and tongue. With the lips closed, the 'M' sound is produced but when open the 'Aah' sound results. (A combination of these two is the easiest modification to make, and it is a possible reason that the word for mother in almost every language in the world is 'muma' or thereabouts.) By holding larynx and lips closed, allowing a little pressure to build up and then releasing them, the 'P' sound results. Repeat this using the tip of the tongue instead of the lips and a 'T' is produced. Thus by using the basic vibration of the larynx, adjusting flow of air over the cords, and altering the volume and shape of the resonating chamber into which the sound projects (pharynx, oral cavity, nasal cavity, and sinuses) the vast variety of sounds that a human being is capable of creating can be produced. The developing child experiments with teeth, tongue, and palate positions, (provided he or she can hear to imitate – deaf children do not acquire speech) and this babbling becomes the basis of speech.

In summary, the functions of the larynx are:

- A rigid conduit for respiratory exchange
- A sphincter mechanism to prevent aspiration
- A reflex protective mechanism (cough)
- A vocal organ
- Fixation of the thorax for effort. Effort such as straining and lifting is more efficient if the glottis is closed and the thorax stable.

11 Structured approach to examination of the throat, head, and neck

The summary in Table 11.1 will assist in an examination of the throat, head, and neck.

Table 11.1 Aids to examination of the throat, head, and neck

General inspection of the head and neck Is there any obvious asymmetry or are there any obvious deformities?
General inspection of the face Is there any obvious bony structural or soft tissue asymmetry or are there any obvious deformities?
Inspection of the lips Is there any abnormality in appearance or of movement?
Assessment of mouth opening Is there any trismus or asymmetrical jaw movement? Are dentures present?
Assessment of the tongue Is there any abnormality of tongue movement or appearance?
Assessment of the oral cavity and visible pharynx Is there any visible abnormality of:

Table 11.1 continued

- the buccal sulcus
- the dental arches
- the floor of the mouth
- the hard and soft palate
- the tonsils and base of tongue
- the visible pharynx?

What additional information is gained from palpation and bimanual palpation?

Palpation of the neck
Are any palpable masses present and if so, what is the site, size, consistency, contour, attachment, and degree of tenderness of any mass?

Step 1

Begin with a general visual inspection of the head and neck.
Does the area appear to be normal or abnormal?

- Asymmetry: consider congenital causes
- Deformities: consider congenital causes, acquired deformities

Pay attention to:

- The parotid area
- The retromandibular area
- The submental area
- The visible, anterior neck above the collar

Are there any obvious deformities, abnormal masses, sores, or scars? If any of these deformities are present, question the patient concerning them, inspect them closely, and bear them in mind for closer examination when examining the neck.

Step 2

Focus in on the face, particularly around the mouth.

Is there facial asymmetry? If this is due to a bony structural asymmetry you can sometimes accentuate this if you place a spatula horizontally between the teeth:

Does the spatula lie horizontally or is it angled? If there is structural asymmetry, consider congenital hemifacial microsomia, acquired maxillary or mandibular deformity. Asymmetry may be the result of a facial nerve palsy. Assess facial muscle movements by asking patients to raise their eyebrows, shut their eyes tight, wrinkle up their nose, show you their teeth. If this is the cause of the asymmetry, consider all the causes of facial nerve palsy.

Are there any obvious deformities, scars, masses, or sores? If present, question the patient concerning these deformities, inspect them closely, including palpation, and initiate thought processes for a differential diagnosis. Bear in mind the possibility of basal cell and squamous cell carcinoma in any ulcerating facial lesions.

Step 3

Ask patients to show you their teeth in order to get them to move the lips apart.

Is there any abnormality of lip movement? If there is any abnormality, then consider facial palsy, scarring, inhibition of movement by trauma, tumour, or inflammatory masses.

Is there any abnormality in the appearance of the lips? Abnormalities include: colour, sores and other ulcerations (benign and malignant), swellings, and traumatic lesions.

If there is any abnormality of movement or appearance, initiate thought processes for a differential diagnosis.

Step 4

Ask patients to open their mouth wide.

Is there any trismus? If there is trismus, consider temporomandibular joint disorders, inflammatory or invasive disorders of the tonsils, pharynx, pterygoid muscles. To examine the temporomandibular joint, place the tips of your index fingers into the conchal bowl of the ears with the pulp facing forwards. Ask patients to open and close their mouth and feel the movements in the joints. Does this cause pain? This may be indicative of temporomandibular joint dysfunction.

Is there asymmetrical movement of the jaw? If there is such movement, consider temporomandibular joint disorders, congenital or acquired mandibular deformity.

Are dentures present? Ask patients to remove them.

Step 5

Ask patients to put out their tongue.

Does it deviate? If it does, consider hypoglossal palsy, invasive disorders of tongue or floor of mouth.

Inspect the surface of the tongue.

Is it normal or abnormal? Abnormal appearances include: smooth, 'hairy', fissured, 'geographic', leukoplakia, ulceration, visible tumours (benign and malignant). Note any abnormalities as you will come back to palpate this area later. In the meantime, initiate thought processes for a differential diagnosis.

Step 6

Ask patients to put their tongue back into their mouth. Using a light and a spatula – two spatulas if you use a headlight:

Examine the buccal sulcus and extend this to the inner aspects of the cheek. Inspect the openings of the parotid ducts. Is the area, in particular the mucosa, normal or abnormal? Abnormalities include: colour, ulceration, 'spots', sloughs/deposits, leukoplakia, masses, pigmented lesions. Initiate thought processes for differential diagnosis.

Examine the dental arches – dentulous/edentulous, caries, gingivitis, gingival ulceration (infection, malignant), alveolar masses. Consider the need for dental referral.

Step 7

Move inside the dental arches, push the tongue out of the way with a spatula, and examine the floor of the mouth anteriorly, laterally, and far back into the 'hidden area'. While here, examine the retromolar trigone area.

Are these areas normal or abnormal? Abnormalities include: ulceration (differential diagnosis of oral ulceration), malignant-looking ulceration or masses, cysts (rannula, cystic hygroma), other masses (haemangioma, impacted stones in submandibular duct). Note any abnormalities as you will come back to palpate this area later.

Step 8

Ask patients to relax their tongue. Inspect the hard palate.

Is it normal or abnormal? Abnormalities include: ulcers (differential diagnosis of oral ulceration including malignant), high arched, cleft palate (scarred, fistula), torus palatinus.

Step 9

Depress the tongue a little and inspect the soft palate/uvula.

Is it normal or abnormal? Abnormalities include: inflamed, swollen, oedematous, ulceration, malignant-looking ulceration, masses, cleft palate, bifid uvula.

Ask patients to say 'Aaah' and observe palatal movement.

Is it normal or abnormal? Abnormalities include bilateral/unilateral paralysis or inhibition of movement by tumour or inflammatory masses.

Step 10

Place the spatula a little further back and depress the tongue. Inspect the base of the tongue, the tonsillar area, and the visible pharynx. Request patients to say 'Aaah' as this makes the tonsils more prominent.

Is the base of tongue normal or abnormal? Abnormalities include: lingual thyroid nodule, cyst in base of tongue, lingual tonsil enlargement.

Are the tonsils absent or present? If present, are they normal or abnormal? Abnormalities include: inflammation (generalized, follicular), enlargement (bilateral or unilateral – the tonsil itself or a mass lateral to the tonsil pushing it medially), slough/membrane, inclusion cysts/bodies, malignant ulceration.

Is the visible pharynx normal or abnormal? Abnormalities include: lymphoid nodules, visible adenoid, postnasal drip, malignant-looking ulceration.

Note any abnormalities for attempted palpation but in the meantime initiate thought processes for a differential diagnosis.

Examination of the deeper areas of the pharynx and the larynx requires special techniques which are not difficult to learn – indirect examination using a mirror or direct examination using a flexible fibre-optic endoscope. In general, when symptoms relate to the hypopharynx/upper oesophagus ('lump in throat', dysphagia) or to the larynx (change in voice, hoarseness), referral for specialist examination is required.

Step 11

If any abnormality had been noted as indicated above, palpate the area at this stage using a gloved index finger to probe around inside the oral cavity.

In the floor of mouth, carry out a bimanual palpation, feeling the tissues between the gloved, intra-oral finger and the fingers of the other hand probing in the submental area. Try and determine the nature of any masses felt – lymph nodes, submandibular salivary gland, Wharton's duct stone, or rannula.

In the tongue, palpation gives a fairly accurate idea as to whether any lesion is superficial or involves the deeper tongue tissues.

In many patients lesions of the tonsils and base of tongue may be palpated as well, although most will gag as you attempt to do this.

Step 12

View the neck with the collar undone, the sternal notch

exposed, and the neck exposed out to the shoulder. Bear in mind any abnormalities noted earlier for closer examination.

Are there any abnormalities, scars, masses that were not seen earlier? Question patients concerning these. Do anterior masses move when you ask them to swallow or put out their tongue? Movement indicates association with the thyroglossal tract and the larynx.

Stand behind patients and palpate the whole of the neck region. Start in the submental area, move back to the submandibular area, then to the retromandibular area. Move up to the parotid area and then back to the upper posterior triangle. Move down the posterior triangle, forwards along the clavicle, and up the posterior aspect of the sternomastoid. Move down the anterior aspect of the sternomastoid, digging your finger tips deep in beneath the muscle. Move up to the hyoid, clasp it gently between index finger and thumb and rock it gently. Move down to the thyroid cartilages, clasp them gently between index finger and thumb, and move them gently sideways and back feeling for laryngeal crepitus as they grate over the cervical spine. Move down and palpate the cricoid cartilage with the tip of the index finger. With both hands try to palpate the thyroid gland on either side and its isthmus centrally (normal glands are impalpable). Palpate the trachea, check that it is central. Finally palpate in the sternal notch.

For any masses felt you need to elucidate the following:

- Site
- Size
- Consistency – hard, firm, rubbery, cystic, soft
- Contour – smooth, irregular
- Attachment – to skin, deeper structures, other structures ('matted')
- Tenderness

With this information, initiate thought processes for a differential diagnosis.

Step 13

Piecing together all the information obtained from the

history regarding patients' throat, head, and neck complaint and the findings on examination as far as you have been able to examine should enable you to make a diagnosis in many cases and initiate treatment. Problems relating to the deeper areas of the pharynx and larynx may require referral for an ENT specialist opinion.

12 Core knowledge of throat, head, and neck disorders

The mouth

Ulcers

The main causes of oral ulceration are:

- Aphthous/herpetic
- Traumatic
- Allergic/auto-immune
- Infective
- Neoplastic

These can usually be distinguished from a combination of the history and examination.

Aphthous/herpetic. Aphthous ulcers tend to be recurrent and are sited predominantly on mobile mucosal surfaces such as the cheek and gingivobuccal sulcus. Herpes ulcers tend to predominate on non-mobile mucosal surfaces such as the hard palate. They both have similar clinical features, usually starting as small vesicles that rapidly ulcerate. They may be of any size and number, are intensely painful but resolve spontaneously over two to three weeks. If any treatment is needed, topical antiseptics/astringents may be used or protective paste applied. Hydrocortisone pellets may be helpful with aphthous ulcers. Acyclovir may be considered for herpes ulcers.

Traumatic. These usually arise from contact with jagged teeth or rough areas on dentures, from biting the cheek or tongue or from other trauma. Apart from removal of the underlying cause, no specific treatment is usually required.

Allergic/auto-immune. Painful ulceration of the oral mucosa is occasionally related to allergy or an auto-immune disease. Some names to remember are:

- Stevens-Johnson syndrome tends to occur in young adults. They present with a maculopapular rash; anal, genital, and oral mucosal ulcers; a fever; headache; and arthralgia. It is thought to be an allergic reaction to foods, drugs, viral, and bacterial infections.
- Behçets syndrome is a combination of iritis, oral and genital ulceration. The cause is unknown.
- Pemphigus is a rare disorder affecting the elderly in which successive crops of blisters occur that heal with scarring.

Treatment of these causes for oral ulceration is non-specific with local, topical therapy supplemented by use of systemic steroids.

Infective. Vitamin deficiencies, particularly vitamin C, may present with infected gingival ulceration.

Haematological disorders (agranulocytosis, leukaemia) often present with infected oral and pharyngeal ulceration.

Vincent's angina – acute ulcerative stomatitis – tends to occur in patients with poor nutrition, low general resistance, and poor oral hygiene. Infection (a combined spirochaete/anaerobic bacterial infection) starts in the gingival margin, spreads and coalesces, and often progresses to cellulitis with swelling of the soft tissue of the floor of mouth. Treatment is with IV penicillin/metronidazole.

Always bear in mind the possibility of TB and syphilis (primary chancre, secondary snail track ulcers, tertiary gumma).

Neoplastic. Always consider malignant neoplastic change when there is persistent ulceration, particularly in tobacco users (smoking, chewing). These are often asymptomatic until infected. They have a typical 'craggy' appearance, usually with hyperkeratosis and infiltration of surrounding soft tissue. Urgent referral is required for biopsy, diagnosis, and treatment.

White/red lesions

Thrush. Candidiasis occurs in the very young, in debilitated adults, in patients on broad-spectrum antibiotics, in patients who are immunocompromised (steroids, immunosuppressants, HIV), and in patients with long-term feeding tubes. Typically the infected mucosa is covered by a white membrane which, when removed, reveals a raw mucosal surface. When arising beneath dentures, the infected area is usually just red and raw. On the lips infection produces raw cracks at the angles (angular cheilitis). Treatment is with topical fungicides as either tablets (pessaries) or solutions.

Leukoplakia. This term is used to describe white plaques of hyperkeratosis on mucosal surfaces. The underlying pathological spectrum ranges from squamous metaplasia through squamous dysplasia to squamous neoplasia. It is usually caused by irritants such as local trauma from teeth or from tobacco usage, but leukoplakia is commonly seen in AIDS patients. Sometimes this same spectrum of pathology may present with predominantly red plaques which are then given the name 'erythroplakia'. Both types of lesion always require biopsy because about 10 per cent will have already progressed to carcinoma in situ by the time they present. In those that have not, resolution frequently follows removal of the irritant. Those that do not resolve require regular follow-up and re-biopsy.

Pigmented lesions

People with naturally pigmented skin may have patchy areas of melanotic pigmentation in the oral mucosa. Peutz-Jeghers syndrome is an association between freckles on the face, patchy pigmentation in the oral mucosa, and gastro-intestinal polyposis. Increased melanin deposition from ACTH stimulation is a feature of Addison's disease – adrenal atrophy – and this may occur on the tongue and in the oral mucosa. Malignant melanoma may also arise in the oral and nasal mucosa.

Swellings

Prominent '**sucking pads**' and **cysts** of dental origin are occasionally seen in infants.

Fibrous traumatic **polyps** occur when the cheek mucosa is repeatedly trapped between teeth or dentures. Treatment involves correction of dentition and surgical excision.

Retention cysts may occur due to obstruction of minor salivary gland ducts. They most frequently occur in the floor of the mouth, when they are known as 'ranula' (*L. rana* = frog). Here they sometimes reach considerable size. Treatment is by surgical marsupialization.

Lymphangioma arises from developmental malformation of lymphatic drainage channels which results in oedematous swelling and deformity of the involved soft tissue – in the oral cavity this may be cheek, lips, tongue, or submandibular area. When multiple cysts form in the involved tissue, the condition is known as **cystic hygroma**. These patients require referral to a specialist service for assessment for surgical excision or debulking as these malformations do not involute spontaneously.

Haemangioma is a similar malformation affecting the vascular channels and is characterized by the bluish discoloration of the swelling. These lesions tend to increase in size over the first year or two of life but usually then involute over the next two to three years. These patients require referral to a specialist service for assessment as surgical excision is sometimes required.

Torus palatinus and **torus mandibularis** are terms used to describe non-neoplastic, localized overgrowths of the underlying bone in these areas. Surgical excision or debulking may be required if the swelling interferes with denture fitting.

Neoplasia. Benign neoplasms of structures beneath the oral mucosa (bone, dental elements, glandular tissue) tend to present as an intra-oral mass. Malignant neoplasia occasionally presents as a swelling rather than an ulcerated lesion. A combination of examination and palpation gives some idea of the extent of the lesion which is best assessed by CT scanning. Patients in whom this is the suspected diagnosis require

R referral to a specialist service for assessment and management.

The tongue

Macroglossia (uncommon) refers to a tongue that is large in relation to the size of the oral cavity and **microglossia** (rare) to one that is small.

Fissured tongue is usually a congenital condition. Debris accumulation can precipitate infection with soreness and halitosis.

Black hairy tongue is caused by overgrowth of filiform papillae and is usually associated with tobacco usage. Treatment is by removal of the irritant, scraping, and brushing.

Geographic tongue is the term used to describe red patches on the tongue surface in which there is an absence of filiform papillae. Characteristically these patches gradually coalesce and change pattern with time. Treatment is not required.

Median rhomboid glossitis refers to a red mass just anterior to the circumvallate papillae which is a remnant of the embryological tuberculum impar. It needs to be distinguished from a **lingual thyroid remnant**. (Remember that if there is lingual thyroid tissue the thyroid gland may have not descended during embryological development and this may be the only functioning thyroid tissue. Sometimes these bleed and surgical excision may be contemplated, in which case a thyroid scan is mandatory.)

Strawberry tongue is the appearance seen in scarlet fever.

Glossitis (painful inflammation) is seen in vitamin B (pellagra) and vitamin C deficiencies.

'Smooth' tongue is seen in iron deficiency anaemia.

The teeth

Dental caries, gingivitis, and associated dental problems are common. Dental-related infection may present as apical abscess, maxillary sinusitis, cellulitis of the cheeks, submandibular cellulitis, or indeed abscess formation anywhere around the face and upper neck. It may also be a cause for lymphadenitis.

An epulis is a granulomatous mass arising between teeth, usually related to pregnancy but also sometimes seen in infants before the teeth have erupted.

A variety of tumours arise from dental elements that present with expansion of the upper or lower jaws.

Edentulous patients, partial or complete, may present with otalgia as a consequence of temporomandibular joint dysfunction. Following removal of teeth, the alveolar ridges gradually atrophy with consequent malocclusion and 'strain' on the TM joint from overclosure during the action of chewing – see Chapter 11, page 140 for how to examine the TM joint when this is a suspected cause of otalgia. When dentures are fitted they need to be adjusted every few years to compensate for this atrophy.

The pharynx

Pharyngitis

Infective. Viral infections are the most common but the infection may be primarily bacterial – usually streptococcal – when there is more systemic upset and more local inflammation than with viral infections. Uncommonly it may be due to candida infection – usually in immunocompromised patients.

Non-infective. Non-infective pharyngitis usually arises from inhalation or ingestion of irritants of which tobacco smoke is the most common. A painful, dry throat is common after radiotherapy.

Tonsillitis

The tonsils form part of a ring of lymphoid tissue around the upper aerodigestive tract – Waldeyer's ring. This is the first site of contact between allergens, organisms, and pathogens and the body immune system. An infant starts life with very little resistance to infection and gradually progresses through childhood to a stage of immunocompetence as contact is made with those things that stimulate the immune system. During this time the tonsils will be continually reacting to each new contact. These episodes of reaction may be regarded as being part of normal development and in most children mean that throughout this period the tonsils will be somewhat enlarged. Occasionally the reaction will be inflammatory in nature, usually associated with a viral pharyngitis, but these minor inflammatory episodes require only symptomatic treatment.

Sometimes the tonsils become acutely inflamed – acute tonsillitis. This happens when bacteria, often streptococcal, which are resident in the tonsil crypts multiply and invade the tonsil stroma to cause infection. The result is an inflammatory swelling of the tonsils with pus discharge from the tonsil crypts, accompanied by fever, systemic upset, and dysphagia. In this situation antibiotics are indicated to both shorten the course of the illness and to reduce the possibility of streptococcal complications (rheumatic fever, glomerulonephritis).

Tonsillectomy is an operation to remove the tonsils and this is indicated for several different reasons:

- Recurrent infection – as a general rule in childhood a tonsillectomy has to be 'earned' since episodes of tonsillitis can generally be treated with antibiotics. The usual indication is when a child has been getting more than four episodes per year for more than two years.
- Persistent infection – this is a different indication and in this state the tonsil infection doesn't resolve with antibiotics. The tonsillitis is either chronic or recurs frequently over a short period of time. This is often the case in adolescents and adults.
- Obstructive sleep – see under *Snoring*, Chapter 8, page 111. The tonsils may not necessarily be inflamed but often enlarge and cause airway obstruction during sleep (the adenoid is often enlarged as well). Tonsillectomy may form

part of the surgery to relieve obstructed sleep, usually in children, but tonsil hypertrophy may be part of the problem in obese adults.

- Suspicion of neoplasia or chronic disease when there is unilateral tonsil enlargement or persistent cervical adenopathy. In these cases the tonsils are removed for histological examination.
- Following a quinsy – see below.

Quinsy

Sometimes during an episode of tonsillitis, an abscess forms in the tonsil bed. This is heralded by the onset of intense pain and dysphagia with spasm of the muscles of mastication causing trismus. When examined, the tonsil pillar and adjacent soft palate are inflamed and swollen, and the tonsil is pushed across to the midline (see Figure 12.1). Relief of the intense pain is achieved by either aspirating or draining the abscess (see *Draining a quinsy* in Chapter 14, page 197) and the infection is treated with intravenous antibiotics. (If general anaesthetic is required for drainage, a 'hot' tonsillectomy may be considered.) Following resolution of the infection tonsillectomy is indicated – see above.

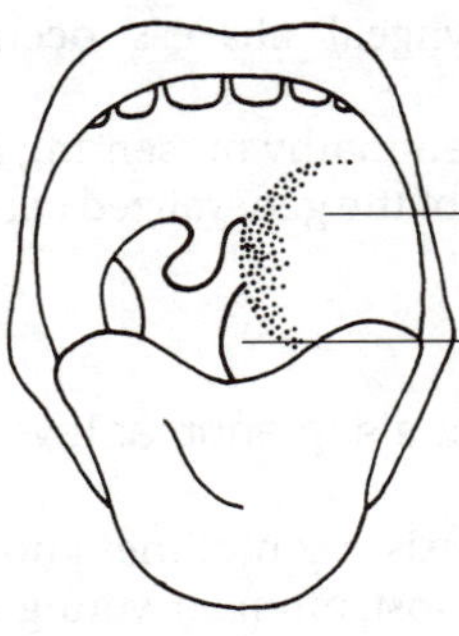

Figure 12.1 Quinsy

Parapharyngeal abscess

When infection of either tonsil or dental origin spreads posteriorly and laterally, an abscess may form in the parapharyngeal space. Here the predominant swelling will be posterior to the tonsil pillars. With enlargement a 'dumb-bell' abscess may form with presentation in the neck as well. It is a potentially serious infection because of the risk of inferior spread to the mediastinum. Treatment is by drainage – internally via the pharynx, externally via the neck – and intravenous antibiotics.

Retropharyngeal abscess

Retropharyngeal abscesses usually occur in infancy when retropharyngeal adenitis progresses to abscess formation. These infants present with fever, systemic upset, and progressive upper airway obstruction. The diagnosis is easily missed until the airway obstruction becomes life-threatening – see *Emergency aspiration of a retropharyngeal abscess,* Chapter 14, page 198. If this diagnosis is suspected and the situation is less urgent, a lateral neck X-ray will show widening of the retropharyngeal soft tissue shadow. The retropharyngeal swelling may be palpated for confirmation. Drainage is undertaken under anaesthetic and the infection treated with intravenous antibiotics.

When a retropharyngeal abscess occurs in an adult, suspect TB.

Retropharyngeal adenopathy presenting as a retropharyngeal mass may be part of the generalized cervical adenopathy of AIDS.

Infectious mononucleosis (glandular fever)

Infectious mononucleosis is sometimes known as the 'kissing disease' and is seen most often in young adults who then present with acute sore throat. When examined the tonsils are inflamed, enlarged, and covered by a membranous exudate (suspect diphtheria when this appearance is seen in infants). There is a marked cervical lymphadenopathy and there may also be hepatosplenomegaly. Atypical lymphocytes are seen in a blood smear (a differential white cell count is mandatory as acute leukaemia sometimes presents with a similar clinical picture) and the Paul-Bunnell titre rapidly rises. Treatment is symptomatic – a skin rash developing when ampicillin is prescribed is virtually diagnostic!

Pharyngeal pouch

These pouches are uncommon but when they do occur they usually arise in late middle-age with a male to female predominance of 4:1. A hernia develops posteriorly through a weakness in the inferior constrictor muscle of the pharynx (Killian's dehiscence), the resulting pouch thus communicates with the pharynx. Food and liquids sometimes enter the pouch to cause the symptoms of dysphagia, gurgling, and regurgitation. The diagnosis is made radiologically (barium swallow) and the treatment is surgical.

Corrosive ingestion

Ingestion of corrosive chemicals is either accidental (usually in children) or suicidal. The corrosive is usually either alkaline (caustic soda) or acid (battery acid) but potassium permanganate may produce deep burns in addition to staining the mucosa brown. Both acids and alkali burn the oral cavity, the pharynx, the larynx, and the oesophagus but acids may burn the stomach and duodenum as well. The burns may only be superficial in areas of rapid transit but tend to be deep in areas of hold-up – at the oesophageal inlet in the pharynx, at the level of the heart in the mid-oesophagus, and at the gastro-oesophageal junction. Superficial burns sometimes heal with minimal scarring (although adhesions may develop between adjacent burnt surfaces) but deep burns heal with fibrosis, which subsequently contracts to cause either stenosis or obliteration of the lumen.

Management is initially concerned with identification of the extent of mucosal injury and any potential complications – laryngeal oedema causing airway obstruction, airway aspiration causing respiratory distress, oesophageal perforation causing mediastinitis, gastric perforation causing peritonitis. This requires endoscopy. A nasogastric feeding tube is then passed both for nutrition and to maintain a lumen. Prophylactic antibiotics are given to combat secondary infection and antacids given to reduce further injury from gastro-oesophageal reflux.

Healing of superficial burns and return of swallowing takes one to two weeks but follow-up is needed to ensure that no dysphagia results from adhesions. Deeper burns take many weeks to heal and invariably regular dilatation of the lumen is required thereafter to reduce the stenosing effect of the healing fibrosis. Occasionally this is unsuccessful, when oesophageal resection with colon replacement becomes necessary.

The larynx

Inflammatory disorders

Laryngitis. Primary infection is usually viral in origin as part of a generalized respiratory tract infection. The exception is epiglottitis – see below. Secondary infection or inflammatory swelling is associated with bacterial infection of either upper or lower respiratory tract. The inflammatory reaction of the laryngeal mucosa (which is exacerbated by coughing) consists of both mucosal induration and oedema within Reinke's space (a potential space between the mucosa and the underlying fibromuscular cord).

In an adult, with a larger larynx than in a child, hoarseness is the predominant symptom of laryngitis, together with pain and irritation (coughing). Treatment of viral infections is symptomatic – steam inhalations may be soothing – but when laryngitis is associated with other bacterial infection antibiotics are recommended. The patient should be told to avoid overuse of the voice as this may prolong resolution of the oedema.

In an infant, laryngitis is a more sinister disorder. It is given the name **laryngo-tracheo-bronchitis (LTB)** which indicates the generalized nature of the infection. Its other name, croup (of Scottish origin), refers to the sound of the typical cough. It tends to affect infants in the ages between six months to three years and starts as a viral respiratory tract infection which gradually worsens into a croupy cough with stridor. Oedema and induration of the laryngeal mucosa predominates, particularly in the immediate subglottic area below the vocal cords. Airway narrowing at this level may progress to total obstruction. Stridor, which is indicative of airway obstruction, becomes the predominant symptom. The difficulty in LTB lies in determining the severity of the obstruction. Perhaps the best guide is to observe the characteristics of the stridor – see *Hoarseness and stridor*, Chapter 13, page 179. Nebulized adrenaline inhalations are given to improve the airway.

In addition to management of the airway, consideration has to be given to use of steroids which, by reducing inflammatory swelling, may reduce the need for airway intervention and shorten the course of the illness. Secondary bacterial, lower respiratory tract infection is common and antibiotics may be needed when the sputum becomes purulent.

Epiglottitis/supraglottitis. This is a primary bacterial infection (*Haemophilus influenzae*) of the supraglottic mucosa. Not common, it is usually seen in children of a slightly older age group than LTB but it also occurs in young adults. It is an even more sinister condition than LTB because of the rapid onset of total laryngeal airway obstruction by the inflamed (cherry red) epiglottis. What begins as a sore throat accompanied by fever and malaise, rapidly progresses to painful dysphagia with stridor and increasing airway obstruction. These patients sit upright with the head and neck rigidly held in one position as they struggle to maintain an airway. Upon presentation, emergency airway intervention (intubation or tracheostomy) is usually required but, if time permits, a lateral neck X-ray will show an enlarged epiglottic shadow. Once the airway is secured, intravenous antibiotics are given (chloramphenicol, cephalosporin) and the infection resolves over four to five days.

Irritants. Exposure to irritants, of which the most potent is tobacco smoke, produces either a non-specific induration/oedema or, of more concern, leukoplakia – see *Neoplasia* on next page. Resolution usually follows removal of the irritant (unless neoplasia has already occurred).

Other causes of laryngeal inflammation include:

- Gastric acid irritation, which occurs with severe gastro-oesophageal reflux, may cause laryngeal mucosal inflammation. Management is of the underlying reflux (antacids, motility agents, surgery).
- Trauma from inhalation of steam, hot air, or flame in burns.
- Trauma from ingestion of corrosives – caustic soda, battery acid – accidental in children, suicidal in adults.
- TB – usually associated with advanced pulmonary TB – causes a granulomatous ulceration of the laryngeal mucosa. Treatment will produce resolution but the fibrosis that results may permanently affect laryngeal function (airway, voice).

Vocal abuse

Acute vocal abuse (screaming, shouting) may precipitate a haematoma of the vocal cord at the contact site in the middle third of the vocal cords.

Chronic vocal abuse may have two effects:

- A localized thickening of the vocal cords at the contact sites – 'singer's' or 'screamer's' nodes
- A generalized oedema of Reinke's space along both vocal cords

Both acute and chronic vocal abuse cause hoarseness. The treatment is cessation of vocal abuse by correction of the speech production disorder – speech therapy can aid in this. Persistent hoarseness despite speech therapy is an indication for surgery to excise nodules or 'strip' away mucosal oedema. The laser is a useful instrument for this type of laryngeal surgery.

Neoplasia

Suspicion of neoplasia should always remain high in patients with persistent hoarseness (the larynx is the most common site for neoplasia in the head and neck) and, because examination of the larynx is a specialized procedure, remember the dictum 'Any hoarseness persisting for more than a month requires urgent referral for specialist examination'.

There a wide spectrum of **benign neoplasms** that arise in the larynx of both adults and children, none of which are common. The symptoms they cause – hoarseness, stridor, airway obstruction – depend on their site and size. They all require specialist referral for evaluation and management.

One that is worth remembering, and it is more strictly a hyperplasia than a neoplasia, is **juvenile recurrent laryngeal papillomatosis**. This is a warty growth caused by infection of the laryngeal mucosa by human papilloma virus. It usually arises in infancy and may be associated with genital tract papillomatosis in the mother (look for it and treat before subsequent pregnancies). Hoarseness and stridor are the symptoms and because of airway obstruction the warty growths require removal. As the name implies, they tend to recur until spontaneous remission ensues after several years (in common with other warts, this is the basis for many patent 'wart cures'). Tracheostomy may be required.

Malignant neoplasms are more common. They are usually squamous carcinomas whose aetiology is smoking and they tend to present in middle- and old-age. As mentioned previously, the pathological progression is squamous metaplasia – squamous dysplasia – squamous neoplasia. (Leukoplakia in the larynx is a potentially premalignant state and always requires biopsy with regular follow-up and repeat biopsy if it does not regress.)

The general principles of management of malignant neoplasia of the larynx include:

- Diagnosis – suspicion, examination, and biopsy
- Assessment – staging (see *Overview of head and neck cancer*, page 167)
- Therapy – radiotherapy, surgery (local excision, partial laryngectomy, total laryngectomy)
- Rehabilitation – oesophageal speech, tracheo-oesophageal fistula with speaking valve
- Follow-up – second primaries, nodal metastasis, distant metastasis

The earlier treatment is begun for laryngeal malignancy, the better the prognosis – hence the importance of early diagnosis. Typically, treated Stage I cancer has a 90 per cent five-year survival, whereas Stage IV has only a 50 per cent five-year survival.

Laryngeal dysfunction

Laryngeal dysfunction implies some impairment of either the sensory nerve supply to the mucosa or the motor nerve supply to the laryngeal muscles. These affect the predominant functions of the larynx as an airway, a sphincter, and a producer of voice.

Sensory loss is probably more common than motor dysfunction although not as commonly diagnosed because it is almost impossible to detect on examination. Reduced sensation impairs the efficient reflex responses that co-ordinate the sphincter action of the larynx and result in choking or aspiration on swallowing (laryngeal incompetence). Loss of sensation may also impair reflexes needed for swallowing and contribute to dysphagia or a feeling of a lump in the throat – a symptom known as 'globus'.

Motor loss (**recurrent laryngeal nerve palsy**) results in the affected vocal cord taking up a position towards the midline of the glottis (there are three muscles for adduction of the cords – sphincter action – but only one muscle for abduction).

Unilateral palsy is more common than bilateral. The left vocal cord is more commonly affected than the right because of the intrathoracic course of the left recurrent laryngeal nerve, a branch of the vagus. Causes include thyroid surgery or malignancy, cardiac surgery, mediastinal nodes (TB), involvement from carcinoma of the bronchus or oesophagus, and many cases that can only be labelled idiopathic – probably some form of viral neuritis. It presents with a breathy hoarseness from inefficient closure of the cords during speech.

Bilateral palsy, in contrast, presents with stridor and airway obstruction because both cords lie paralysed in the midline. Causes include hydrocephalus, base of skull lesions, congenital mediastinal vessel anomalies, and sometimes cardiac surgery when dissection around the right subclavian artery has been needed to place an arterial line. Many cases, however, can only be labelled idiopathic.

Patients with suspicion of recurrent laryngeal nerve palsy require referral for specialist evaluation.

Other laryngeal disorders

Hypothyroidism. Chronic oedema of the vocal cords (myxoedema) may cause hoarseness.

Angioneurotic oedema. An alarming manifestation of a type I allergic reaction that may rapidly progress to fatal airway obstruction from generalized laryngeal oedema. First aid – give adrenaline by subcutaneous injection and intubate.

Rheumatoid arthritis. The crico-arytenoid joint – the basis for vocal cord movement – may be involved in this disorder when fixity of the cords causes airway obstruction requiring tracheostomy.

Foreign bodies. If large, these will cause total airway obstruction. Small people can be turned upside down and thumped on the back. If this does not dislodge the object, resort to Heimlich's manoeuvre. If not dislodged by this, you will have to perform an emergency tracheostomy – see *Securing an emergency airway* in Chapter 14, page 199. Smaller foreign bodies not causing total obstruction require urgent anaesthetic and removal.

The head and neck

Neck lumps

Neck lumps may arise from:

- The skin and subcutaneous tissues
- Congenital remnants
- The thyroid gland
- The salivary glands
- Bony and cartilaginous structures
- Blood vessels
- Lymph nodes

The skin and subcutaneous tissue

Sebaceous cysts and lipomas are readily identified by the ability to lift up the lump in the skin. If required, treatment is by surgical excision.

Congenital remnants

Frequently these do not present until adolescence or early adulthood.

- **Dermoid cysts** usually present as midline, submental swellings but may occur along any of the other lines of embryological fusion.
- **Thyroglossal cysts** may present anywhere in the midline along the line of embryological descent of the thyroid from base of tongue to the thyroid gland but are most commonly situated either just above or just below the hyoid bone. Classically they move upward with protrusion of the tongue. Usually painless, they may become inflamed with

infection. Abscess formation with discharge may result in a chronic discharging sinus. Treatment involves surgical excision of the cyst and its tract – the mid-portion of the hyoid bone has to be removed as well to prevent recurrence behind it.

- **Branchial cysts** are classically situated beneath the middle third of the sternomastoid muscle and protrude anterior to the muscle (second branchial arch). Usually painless, they can become inflamed because of their association with lymphoid tissue. Treatment involves surgical excision and this can be complicated if there is a tract that travels from the cyst, between the carotid arteries, to terminate in the tonsil.
- **Cystic hygroma** is one presentation of a lymphangioma (abnormality of lymphatic vessels) in which cystic spaces (remember transillumination) enlarge within the soft, irregular mass of tissue that results from impaired lymphatic drainage. Present at birth, they usually enlarge and (unlike haemangioma) do not involute so that surgical excision is required – an extremely difficult procedure as the malformation is diffuse throughout all the involved soft tissues.

Thyroid gland

The thyroid gland is normally impalpable so that all thyroid enlargements are pathological. They move upwards with both tongue protrusion and swallowing. Remember that clinically a patient may be thyrotoxic, euthyroid, or hypothyroid; thyroid function tests may be required and the gland may require to be 'scanned' for radio-active isotope uptake.

- Whole gland enlargement:
  - physiological in adolescents
  - multinodular goitre – one lobe may be more enlarged than the other
  - Hashimoto's disease – auto-immune thyroiditis
- Solitary nodules:
  - benign cysts
  - adenomas
  - malignancy

These are differentiated by isotope scan, needle aspiration for cytology and biopsy.

The salivary glands

The **parotid gland** extends behind the angle of the mandible – swellings here can be confused with lymph nodes. There is also a deep lobe – swellings here may present in the pharynx in the region of the tonsil. The gland is normally impalpable and all swellings are pathological.

- Acute swellings:
  - Mumps – bilateral, painful, diffuse enlargement. Be aware of complications (orchitis, pancreatitis, deafness).
  - Bacterial parotitis – uncommon, usually in the debilitated, dehydrated elderly, it usually presents as a unilateral, painful inflammatory swelling with purulent discharge from the duct orifice. Treatment requires rehydration, IV antibiotics, and drainage if there is any abscess formation.
- Intermittent swellings:
  - Calculi. Large calculi obstructing Stensen's duct are uncommon. The parotid gland swells whenever there is increased salivation (thought and taste of food) and this is painful. They require surgical removal. Smaller calculi obstruct the ductal system within the gland and cause distal dilatation (sialectasis) which is diagnosed by injection of radio-opaque dye (sialogram). If troublesome these glands require total excision (parotidectomy).
  - Auto-immune disease is uncommon but when it does occur it affects middle-aged women more than men. One example is Sjögren syndrome – intermittent, painless, bilateral parotid swelling, dry eyes, and rheumatoid arthritis. The associated dry mouth is known as xerostomia. Lymphoma may develop as a late complication.
- Persistent swellings:
  - Neoplasia, a persistent, unilateral parotid swelling, is invariably neoplastic. Ninety per cent are benign adenomas for which the surgery is 'superficial' parotidectomy (not a simple lumpectomy because of the high recur-

rence rate). Pain and facial nerve palsy are indicators of malignancy but these generally occur late and diagnosis is made either by needle aspiration cytology or by histology. When malignant, these tumours have a low sensitivity to radiotherapy and therefore total parotidectomy is required with sacrifice and grafting of the facial nerve.

The submandibular gland

- Inflammatory swelling secondary to infection in the oral cavity is related to the close association with lymphoid tissue.
- Calculi are more common than in the parotid gland.
- Neoplasia is more likely to be malignant than in the parotid gland.

Bony and cartilaginous structures

Normal structures may be mistaken for pathological lumps, for example transverse process of axis, hyoid bone, thyroid and cricoid cartilages, and accessory cervical rib.

Blood vessels

- Carotid pulsations are palpable but not the artery itself unless thickened by atherosclerosis – remember to listen for a bruit.
- Carotid body tumours (chemodectoma) are rare and arise in the carotid bifurcation. They are pulsatile with an audible bruit.
- In some people the external jugular vein may massively enlarge with straining or when there is mediastinal obstruction.

Lymph nodes

There are more than a hundred lymph nodes on each side of the neck with several named groups of nodes and a definite pattern of drainage. Supraclavicular nodes also drain from the thorax and on the left side (thoracic duct) from the abdomen. (See Figure 12.2.) Inflammatory reaction with enlargement in regional lymph nodes is a normal response to inflammation/infection in the upper aerodigestive tract but should settle as the inflammation/infection resolves or responds to treatment. Persistent palpable, painless lymph node enlargement is normal in childhood but in adults a persistently palpable node should be investigated to exclude a primary underlying neoplasia.

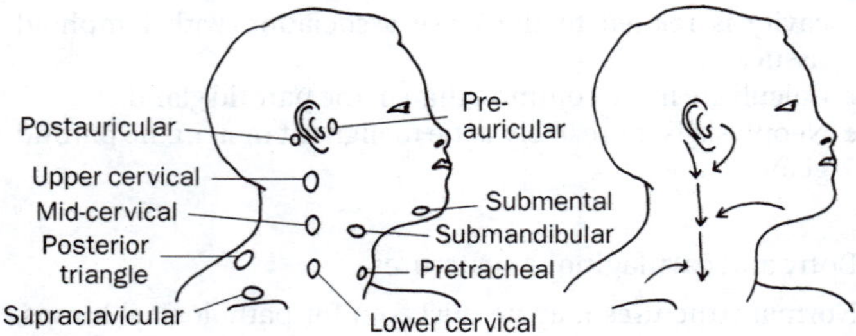

Figure 12.2 Cervical lymph nodes

- **Lymphadenitis** is lymph node enlargement due to inflammation and is usually painful at some stage. Occasionally frank infection may establish in a node and progress to cellulitis and abscess formation.
- **Lymphadenopathy:**
  - Consider infectious mononucleosis – see page 154 – in adolescents with significant, multiple, bilateral nodes. Other body nodes may be involved and there may be hepatosplenomegaly.
  - Consider TB for persistent cervical lymphadenopathy.
  - Persistent, generalized lymphadenopathy is an early feature of HIV infection.
- **Neoplastic lymphadenopathy** – remember the 80:20 rule – see Chapter 13, page 183.
  - Lymphoma, usually Hodgkin's, occurs in both children and adults. It presents with either an isolated node swelling or as a unilateral lymphadenopathy.
  - Metastatic neoplasia – remember the general rule that

any neck lump appearing for the first time in an adult over 40 years of age (20:40 rule) should be regarded as metastatic neoplasia until proven otherwise. Remember also that the prognosis for survival is markedly decreased if a metastatic node is biopsied. Therefore, on suspicion of a metastatic node a search for the primary site of the neoplasm should be made – usually this will be a squamous carcinoma of the upper aerodigestive tract but other malignancies do occur. If not obvious, urgent referral to a specialist service is mandatory for primary site identification and biopsy. If the primary site cannot be identified, needle aspiration for cytology or needle biopsy are preferred to open biopsy of the neck node. Management of metastatic neoplastic disease involves management of the primary site together with a radical neck dissection in which all likely metastatic node-containing tissue in the drainage area is excised.

Overview of head and neck cancer

The head and neck region is a common site for cancer, and malignancy in the upper aerodigestive tract accounts for 15 to 20 per cent of all cancer. In this region both the cancerous lesion and any surgery required for treatment affect eating, drinking, speaking, and respiration as well as producing cosmetic deformity with its associated psychological effects. On the brighter side, malignancy tends to remain confined to the primary site and its regional nodes, with distant metastasis usually a late event. Local treatment with radiotherapy and surgery, especially if the cancer is identified early, offers reasonable prospect of cure. Typically, patients with treated Stage 1 cancers have a better than 75 per cent chance of five-year survival.

The majority of cancers arising from mucosal surfaces are squamous carcinoma. Often the onset of malignancy is preceded by leukoplakia or erythroplakia and in these lesions a histological progression of disease may be recognized – squamous metaplasia, squamous dysplasia, carcinoma in situ, frank carcinoma. Alcohol and tobacco (smoked, chewed, or inhaled as snuff) appear to act synergistically as the predominant aetiological factors for development of squamous carcinoma. Some of the other cancers encountered in the head and neck have known aetiological factors:

- Adenocarcinoma arising within the sinuses has been associated with long-term exposure to hardwood dust in woodworkers.
- Sarcomas and thyroid malignancies are associated with previous radiation exposure.
- Immunocompromised patients (immunosuppressants, HIV infection) may develop non-Hodgkin's lymphomas, squamous cell carcinomas, or Kaposi's sarcoma.
- Epstein Barr virus is linked to carcinoma of the nasopharynx and Burkitt's lymphoma.

The principles of management of malignancy in this area are:

1. **Diagnosis**. Examination and biopsy of the primary site – see *Neoplastic lymphadenopathy*, page 166.
2. **Assessment:**
    - Identification of the primary site.
    - Determination of the extent of disease at the primary site by inspection, palpation, CT and MRI scanning, and hence staging – see below.
    - Identification of nodal metastasis by palpation with needle aspiration for cytology.
    - Determination of the extent of nodal disease by palpation, CT and MRI scanning, and hence staging.
    - Identification of distant metastasis.

From this information, the patient's cancer is staged according to a staging classification known as the TNM system:

T = Primary tumour. T0, T1 to T4. The exact description of each T stage differs for the various anatomical sites.
N = Nodes. N0, N1 to N3.
M = Distant Metastasis. M0 or M1.

3. **Formulation of treatment plan**. This is largely determined by the staging of primary disease and nodal metastases. In

this region distant metastasis renders the disease incurable.

- Early stage disease – radiotherapy with the option of salvage surgery for radiation failure.
- Later stage disease – a combination of surgical ablation and radiotherapy.
- Late stage disease:
  - potentially curable – a combination of chemotherapy, radiotherapy, and surgical ablation
  - incurable – palliative chemotherapy and/or radiotherapy, terminal care.

4. **Rehabilitation**. Surgical ablation and reconstruction produces not only cosmetic but functional disability. Rehabilitation of swallowing and speaking are usually required.
5. **Follow-up**. Recurrence of disease is most likely to manifest within the first two to three years after treatment and thereafter becomes less and less likely. After a five-year disease-free interval the cancer is regarded as cured.
   - Salvage surgery may be possible for disease recurrence detected early.
   - Second-site primary disease will arise in about 15 to 20 per cent of head and neck cancer patients – particularly if the aetiological factors persist. This may be within the same region, in the lower respiratory tract or, perhaps surprisingly, within the lower gastro-intestinal tract.
   - Distant metastasis, although not common, is an ever-present concern, the usual sites being the lungs and liver.

ENT aspects of head and neck trauma

Head injury without skull fracture

Closed head injury may cause avulsion of the olfactory (1st) nerve at the cribriform plate with loss of the sense of smell. This will be permanent.

Similar injury may affect the cochleovestibular (8th) nerve (rare) as it leaves the brain stem to enter the internal auditory canal causing deafness and vertigo. Deafness will be permanent but loss of balance usually compensates with time. (Occasionally there is some recovery of hearing, in which case it is assumed that the nerve was only stretched and not avulsed.)

Whiplash injury to the cervical spine often causes imbalance.

Head injury with skull fracture

Frontal bone. Fractures extending to the cribriform plate or into the frontal sinuses open a tract for cerebrospinal fluid leak. (Remember that CSF can be detected by the presence of glucose when tested with a Dextrostix.) Spontaneous closure usually occurs but there is potential for intracranial spread of infection from the nose – prophylactic antibiotics. Persistent CSF leaks require surgery.

Petrous portion of the temporal bone (base of skull fracture). Fracture lines frequently involve the roof of the middle ear and tear the tympanic membrane – hence bleeding from the ear may be indicative of a base of skull fracture (it may also occur from lacerations of the external canal skin). CSF leak may not be noticed when mixed with blood but can be detected by the halo sign on the ear dressing. As above, spontaneous closure is usual but prophylactic antibiotics are required. This injury frequently disrupts the middle ear – if the deafness is purely conduction, middle ear surgery is warranted. Fracture lines also disrupt the inner ear – sensorineural deafness and vertigo. The facial nerve canal may be disrupted – facial nerve palsy – in which case surgical exploration is required with an attempt to repair the nerve.

Facial fractures

Nasal bones – see *Nasal trauma*, Chapter 8, page 108.

Mandible. Potential sites for fracture are the neck, the angle, the body, or the symphysis; see Figure 12.3. Clinically, jaw movement is limited by reflex muscle spasm, there is haemorrhage from the fracture site with localized tenderness, and the teeth are usually displaced out of alignment.

The fracture is reduced and immobilized by wiring the upper and lower teeth together and sometimes additional plating of the fracture line may be required.

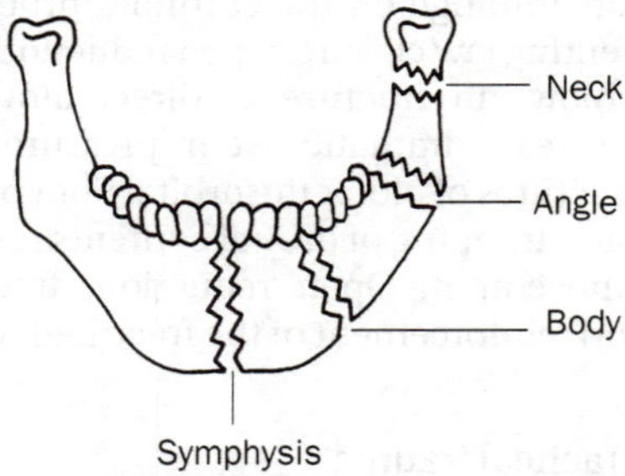

Figure 12.3 Fractures of the mandible

Maxilla. Three classical fracture lines were described by Le Fort (see Figure 12.4) and severe facial trauma may result in any combination of these with posterior displacement. Severe haemorrhage and fatal airway obstruction complicates this type of injury. Management initially involves securing an airway followed later by fracture reduction and fixation with a combination of internal, external, and interdental fixation.

Malar bones. Fractures following a direct blow are usually depressed with a 'step' in the orbital margin and may disrupt the infra-orbital nerve. Open reduction is required with internal fixation.

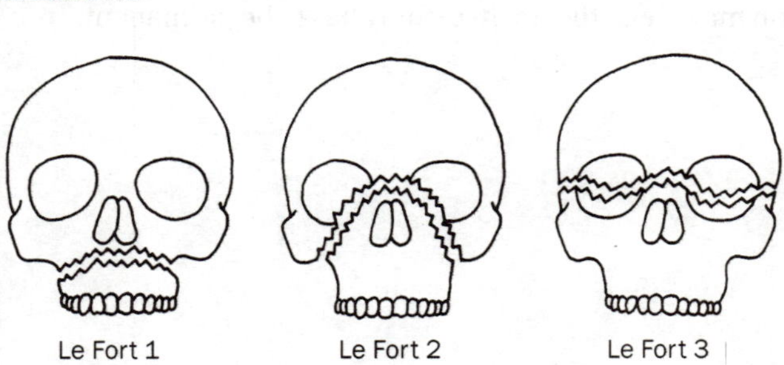

Figure 12.4 Fractures of the facial skeleton

Zygomatic arch. Fractures following a direct blow are usually multiple and depressed. Movement of the underlying temporalis muscle may be affected, causing trismus, or the fracture may impinge on the coronoid process of the mandible, preventing jaw closure. Open reduction is required.

Orbital blow-out fracture. A direct blow to the orbital contents causes a dramatic rise in pressure that may cause blow-out fractures of either the orbital floor or its medial wall. Extrusion and trapping of orbital contents result in limitation of globe movement. Open reduction, freeing of trapped content, and reinforcement of the fractured wall is required.

Laryngo-tracheal trauma

The cartilaginous skeleton of the larynx in children is usually flexible and does not fracture but the internal soft tissues may be disrupted. The adult skeleton is more rigid and subject to fracture dislocation. Clinically, trauma may produce any combination of bleeding, stridor, dysphonia, painful dysphagia, and surgical emphysema. Airway obstruction necessitates emergency tracheostomy (see *Securing an emergency airway* in Chapter 14, page 199), as it may be impossible to pass an endotracheal tube. Once the airway is secured, examination can be undertaken and surgical exploration with repair contemplated. Healing involves fibrosis and invariably there will be persistent hoarseness. Sometimes the fibrosis contracts into a stricture and the consequent airway obstruction may mean the tracheostomy has to be permanent.

13 A practical approach to throat, head, and neck disorders

As mentioned earlier, patients do not usually complain of a specific disorder or disease, but rather complain about their symptoms and discomforts. Disorders causing symptoms and signs relating to the head and neck may be obvious – swellings, inflammation, or trauma – but often the site of the primary pathology is in the throat. In the throat, disorders may have localized symptoms but sometimes these are referred, particularly otalgia. The head, the neck, and the oral cavity can be readily examined but when pathology is situated deeper in the aerodigestive tract, specialist referral will probably be needed to adequately examine the nasopharynx, the pharynx, and the larynx.

Symptoms

The type of complaints from disorders in this region that are likely to bring patients for consultation include:

- Pain
- Dysphagia
- Ingested foreign body
- Problems of salivation
- Hoarseness and stridor
- Neck lump
- Head and neck trauma

A practical approach to disorders in this region starts with trying to make a diagnosis through consideration of the symptoms expressed and findings on examination. The cause may be identified and appropriate treatment for the problem may then be initiated. A precise diagnosis may not be possible if the site of possible pathology cannot be seen. R When this is the case, an appropriate specialist referral will be necessary.

Pain

Pain in the throat, head, and neck is a common problem. The anatomical structures in this area are all supplied by either the 5th cranial nerve – sensory to the skin of the face, neck, and ear; the mucosa of the nose, sinuses and oral cavity; the anterior tongue; and to the teeth – or the 9th and 10th cranial nerves – sensory to the pharynx; the posterior tongue; the larynx; the eustachian tube; and the middle ear. To complicate the problem of pain it can either be localized to the site of disorder or referred to other areas of distribution of the nerves.

The approach to pain therefore involves first a good history regarding the nature and characteristics of the pain to try and separate out facial pain and sore throats from sinusitis and other types of head and neck pain. This is then followed by a careful examination to identify or exclude any disease or disorder that could possibly be the cause for the pain.

Potential causes

Diseases and disorders that have to be considered include:

Sore throat:
- Tonsillitis/pharyngitis.
- Oral and pharyngeal disease – ulcers, infection, tumour (benign and malignant).
- Dental disorders – caries, erupting or impacted teeth, gingivitis, temporomandibular joint dysfunction.
- Malignant disease – an ever-present worry particularly in

tobacco users (smoking, chewing, sniffing). Remember particularly the 'red flag' situation of sore throat with otalgia.

Sinusitis:
See Chapter 9, pages 119-120 for consideration of this type of pain.

Others:

- Localized inflammation from a variety of causes:
  - superficial – minor injury, insect bites, cellulitis, impetigo and other ulceration, shingles
  - deeper seated – cervical adenitis, infection in congenital cysts (branchial, thyroglossal, pre-auricular), dental abscess, other abscesses
- Cervical osteo-arthritis and muscle spasm
- Neuralgias:
  - trigeminal, glossopharyngeal, postherpetic
  - headaches – migraine, cluster, tension, temporal arteritis
  - atypical

Treatment

Having done your best to exclude any of these diseases or disorders there will still be a substantial proportion of patients for whom the cause can only be labelled idiopathic. R Referral for specialist opinion is warranted if there is suspicion of an underlying disease or disorder that you have not been able to exclude.

Dysphagia

Potential causes

Dysphagia may be caused by any of the diseases or disorders of the mouth, pharynx, larynx, or oesophagus. These are discussed in Chapter 12, *Core knowledge of throat, head, and neck disorders.* Classically, painful dysphagia (odynophagia – Greek odyne = pain) is distinguished from painless dysphagia, the former usually indicative of an inflammatory pathology. A good history provides many clues as to the nature of the underlying disorder and examination of the oral cavity should identify disease in this area. Specialist referral is required for adequate examination of the pharynx, larynx, and oesophagus. This will often be supplemented by the mainstay of investigation of dysphagia, the barium swallow.

Even after this there will remain many patients with dysphagia – particularly those with symptoms such as 'difficulty getting the food back and down' or 'a feeling of a lump in the throat' – for which no obvious disease will be found. The term 'globus' is often given to these types of dysphagia. Since swallowing is a complex mechanism involving the co-ordinated contraction and relaxation of something like 20 different muscles, it is probable that the cause is some inco-ordination of the mechanism. Inco-ordination as a cause is obvious when the disorder is gross as in bulbar palsy or cerebral palsy. The cause for the minor degrees of inco-ordination may lie in either the afferent (sensory) or the efferent limb of the neural pathways. Efferent problems are sometimes detected on examination or investigation but afferent problems are almost impossible to detect clinically, which explains why precise diagnosis is difficult when dealing with globus.

Treatment

Treatment of dysphagia is determined by the nature and extent of identified disease or disorder.

It is as well to remember that complications sometimes arise from disease causing dysphagia that may also require attention and these include:

- weight loss, dehydration, cachexia
- aspiration into the lower airway
- perforation of the oesophagus with mediastinitis, a potentially fatal infection

Ingested foreign body

The common sites for impaction of swallowed foreign bodies are the tonsils, the base of the tongue, the pharynx, the oesophageal inlet, or within the oesophagus.

In the oral cavity and the visible oropharynx, localization is good and it should be possible to see and remove the foreign body. In the pharynx, localization is still quite good, but this is a more difficult area to examine and may require use of ENT mirrors or anaesthetic laryngoscopes. Knowing where to concentrate on looking aids identification of a foreign body and radiology may be helpful if the foreign body is radio-opaque. These foreign bodies can often be removed without the need for a general anaesthetic, although the services of an ENT specialist may be required to do this. Sometimes the foreign body may injure the mucosa before passing on and the feeling of impaction may persist. If the foreign body cannot be seen on mirror, direct, or radiological examination, then expectant management may be employed. If there is indeed no foreign body, the sensation should settle over a few hours. If the sensation persists or gets worse, it is probable that the foreign body was missed on examination, and examination under general anaesthesia will be needed to find or exclude it.

Once the foreign body is in the oesophagus, patients have difficulty localizing the site, feeling the sensation in the midline at the level of the larynx. If movement of the larynx exacerbates the sensation, this localizes the site of impaction to the oesophageal inlet. Dysphagia is common in oesophageal impaction and may include inability to swallow even saliva – salivary pooling in the hypopharynx is one clinical sign of impaction. Radiology is helpful if the foreign body is radio-opaque. Oesophageal foreign bodies generally require an anaesthetic for removal. For this reason, if the object is not obstructing, is not sharp, and is not potentially corrosive (for example button batteries), it is reasonable to wait until the next day to see whether it will pass spontaneously into the stomach.

There should always be suspicion of a stricture or a tumour

in adults who have had a foreign body impact in the oesophagus and, if oesophagoscopy was not performed, a barium swallow should be performed before discharging the patient.

Problems of salivation

Disorders of the salivary glands themselves – inflammation, calculi, neoplasia – are discussed in Chapter 12, pages 164-165, salivation problems being considered here.

Salivation associated with dysphagia indicates the severity of the underlying disorder and requires an urgent diagnosis and initiation of appropriate treatment. Examples would include:

- Salivation after ingestion of a corrosive substance by children is the cardinal sign that there has been a significant burn of the mucosa of the mouth, pharynx, or oesophagus
- Salivation after recent onset of sore throat and hoarseness/stridor is a strong indicator that the underlying disorder is epiglottitis – see below
- Salivation after ingestion and impaction of a foreign body indicates total obstruction of the oesophagus – see above

Inadequate salivation: The combined secretions from both the major and minor salivary glands produce a mixture of mucoid and serous saliva, the former having a lubricating and the latter a moisturizing function as well as containing the salivary enzymes. The combined reserve secreting capacity is such that diminution in secretion is not noticeable unless it involves all the glands. This may occur as a side-effect of medication, following radiotherapy and, rarely, in such conditions as auto-immune disease of salivary glands (sicca syndrome).

Drooling in children: Persistent drooling of saliva results not so much from an overall increase in production as from inability to adequately swallow the volume produced. This is seen particularly in patients with cerebral palsy. Medication to reduce salivary flow soon runs into the problem of tachyphylaxis. There are two surgical options, either to denervate the glands (remember that the nerves containing secretomotor fibres to the salivary glands run through the ear – tympanic plexus, chorda tympani) or to re-route the salivary gland ducts so that salivary flow is directed into the pharynx where there is a better chance that it will be swallowed. These surgical procedures, either alone or in combination, can do much to relieve the distress caused by continuous drooling.

Hoarseness and stridor

Hoarseness and stridor are the two cardinal symptoms of laryngeal disorders. There is a fundamental difference between these disorders when they occur in children compared with when they occur in adults. This relates to the size of the airway. In the small airway, disorders will predominantly manifest as airway obstruction and voice changes will be a secondary consideration. In the larger airway, voice disorders will predominate with airway obstruction being a late manifestation of disease.

A good history provides many clues but examination is needed to make a diagnosis. Generally this will require specialist referral.

Regarding hoarseness the cardinal rule is that 'any hoarseness persisting for more than a month requires referral for a diagnosis'. This is because of the ever-present worry that it may be caused by neoplasia, usually benign in children but malignant in adults.

Potential causes

Causes for hoarseness include:

In children:
- Laryngitis – usually laryngo-tracheo-bronchitis (LTB or croup) in infancy
- 'Screamer's' nodes
- Congenital – laryngeal web, laryngeal cyst

- Recurrent laryngeal nerve palsy
- Laryngeal papillomatosis

In adults:

- Laryngitis – acute and chronic
- Vocal abuse – 'singer's' nodes, chronic oedema
- Neoplasia
- Recurrent laryngeal nerve palsy
- Myxoedema

When stridor – which is the clinical sign of airway obstruction – is the presentation, urgent or emergency referral, dictated by the degree of obstruction, is required. In severe cases first aid measures may be necessary while awaiting transfer:

- Attempt to dislodge foreign bodies (digital, laryngoscopic, Heimlich's manoeuvre)
- Nebulized adrenaline inhalations for inflammatory swelling
- Intubation or tracheostomy

Causes for stridor include:
In children:

- Laryngo-tracheo-bronchitis (LTB or croup) – see below
- Epiglottitis – rapid onset of obstruction – see below
- Congenital:
  - variable stridor: laryngomalacia
  - fixed stridor: laryngeal web, laryngeal cyst
- Foreign body
- Laryngeal papillomatosis

In adults:

- Neoplasia
- Bilateral recurrent laryngeal nerve palsy
- Rheumatoid arthritis with crico-arytenoid joint fixation
- Trauma
- Foreign body

Laryngo-tracheo-bronchitis and **epiglottitis** require special mention because they are not uncommon in infants. Of the two conditions, LTB is by far the most common.

Laryngo-tracheo-bronchitis tends to affect a younger age group (6 to 18 months) and the precipitating viral respiratory tract infection gradually worsens into a croupy cough with stridor. The difficulty in LTB lies in determining the severity of the obstruction. Perhaps the best guide is to observe the characteristics of the stridor – see Figure 13.1.

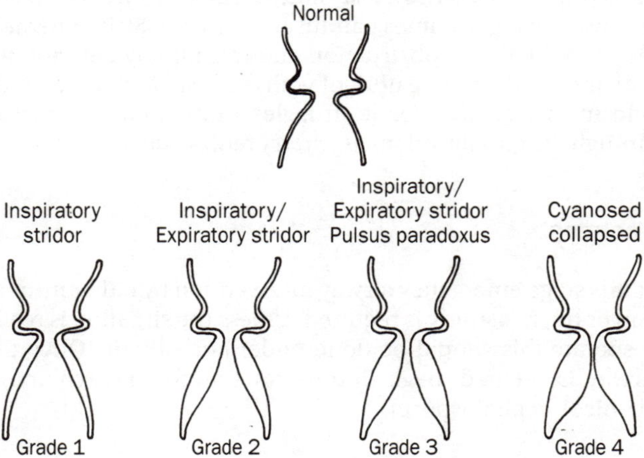

Figure 13.1 Laryngo-tracheo-bronchitis

Treatment

Consideration needs to be given to the use of systemic steroids in all children with LTB.

Grade 1: Inspiratory stridor – minor degree of obstruction – give nebulized adrenaline inhalations.

Grade 2: Inspiratory and expiratory stridor – obstruction is progressing to the stage of requiring intervention – continue nebulized adrenaline but observe closely.

Grade 3: Inspiratory plus expiratory stridor with a palpable pulsus paradoxus (a huge negative pressure is being generated by the inspiratory efforts which affects venous return and hence cardiac output) – airway intervention required by either intubation or tracheostomy under the controlled circumstances of an anaesthetic.

Grade 4: Cyanosis – almost too late – emergency airway intervention required.

Epiglottitis, on the other hand, tends to affect a slightly older age group (two to three years). What starts as a sore throat rapidly becomes a toxic illness. The sore throat worsens and swallowing becomes painful and difficult. Stridor heralds the onset of airway obstruction and this rapidly deteriorates until the child is sitting upright with the head and neck rigidly held in one position as it struggles to maintain an airway through the grossly inflamed (cherry red), swollen epiglottis.

Treatment

At this stage emergency airway intervention by either intubation or tracheostomy is required. Unless the situation is really desperate this should be done under anaesthetic. Once the airway is secured, begin intravenous antibiotics (chloramphenicol, cephalosporin).

Neck lump

Details of the possible structures in the neck that may give rise to lumps are given in Chapter 12 and details of their examination given in Chapter 11. Remember that when a malignancy is suspected the primary site needs to be identified. In a practical approach there are two general rules that may be usefully applied.

The first is the '20:40' rule that applies to the age of the patient:

Less than 20 years:
- Inflammatory neck nodes
- Congenital lesions – thyroglossal cyst, branchial cyst, midline dermoid, cystic hygroma, haemangioma
- Lymphoma

20 to 40 years:
- Chronic infection – HIV, TB
- Salivary gland pathology – calculus, infection, tumour
- Thyroid pathology – goitre, tumour, thyroiditis
- Lymphoma

Older than 40 years:
- Metastatic or primary malignant disease

The second is the '80:20' rule that applies to neoplastic disease presenting as a neck lump. In children, 80 per cent will be benign and isolated but 20 per cent will be malignant. In adults, 80 per cent will be malignant – most commonly metastatic nodes from primary squamous carcinoma of the upper aerodigestive tract – and only 20 per cent will be benign.

Once the cause for this neck lump has been identified, the appropriate treatment can be given – see Chapter 12.

Head and neck trauma

First aid principles of trauma resuscitation apply at the site of first contact with head and neck trauma – secure the airway, control bleeding, etc. Remember that concussive injury to the skull and dislocating injury to the cervical spine may be part of trauma to the head and neck. Once the situation is stable, individual sites of injury may be examined and are broadly classified as open (superficial, deep, or penetrating), or closed.

Areas of ENT involvement in head and neck trauma are discussed in Chapter 12, page 169. In general, further investigation of these areas will be required to determine the full extent of injury and the type of treatment likely to be involved. These investigations are tailored to the particular injury but include:
- Radiology – plain films, contrast studies, CT scan
- Endoscopy – nasal cavities, pharynx, larynx, trachea, oesophagus

- Audiometry for injuries with hearing impairment
- Facial nerve conduction studies for injuries causing facial nerve palsy

Treatment

The structures involved and the extent of injury determine management and this may be either immediate intervention, delayed intervention, or expectant management.

PART IV
ENT skills

14 Practical skills in ENT

Dry mopping of ears

The most commonly used method of cleaning ears that are discharging is by dry mopping; see Figure 14.1. To do this you first have to prepare the mop. Take an orange stick and some cotton wool. Tease out a small piece of cotton wool and place the tip of the orange stick halfway onto it. By twisting the orange stick around and around, wrap the piece of cotton wool onto the end of the stick so that about half of the cotton wool sticks out from the end as a fluffy tip. The size of the fluffy tip is determined by the size of the ear canal into which you are going to insert it. It needs to be thin for a child's ear but can be larger for a wide adult ear canal.

You need to do the actual mopping in good light so that you can see what you are doing. Adults can be mopped while they

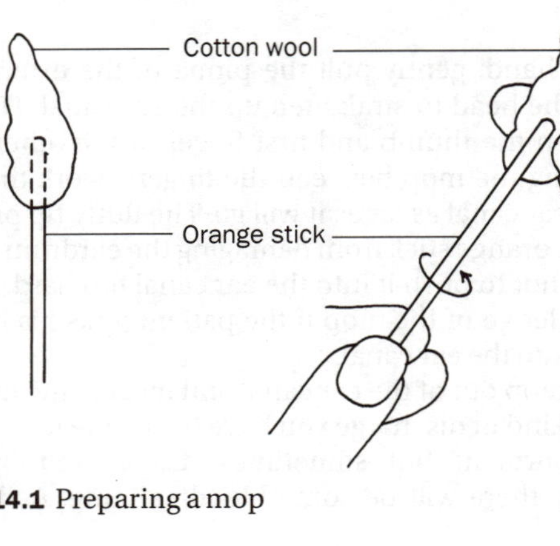

Figure 14.1 Preparing a mop

are sitting sideways-on in front of you with their ear pointing towards the source of light. Children need to wrapped up and held firmly in a sitting position on an adult's lap with one of the adult's hands holding the child's head steady against her body and the other hand holding the child's body so that he can't wriggle; see Figure 14.2. If this is unsatisfactory, the child needs to be laid down on his side on a bed with the ear to be cleaned facing upwards and an adult holding both the child's head and body steady.

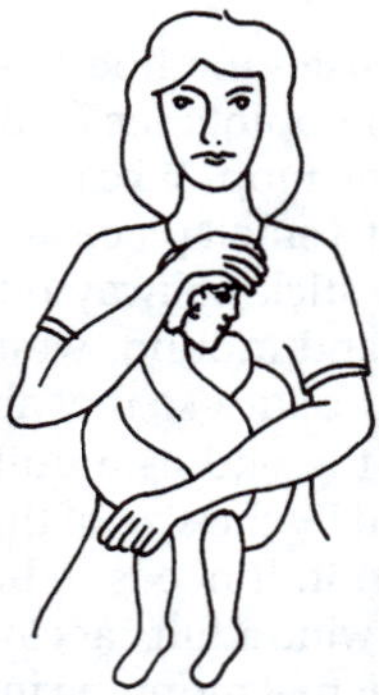

Figure 14.2 Wrapping up and holding a child for ear procedure

With one hand, gently pull the pinna of the external ear away from the head to straighten up the ear canal. Hold the mop between the thumb and first finger of the other hand. While rotating the mop between the fingers, work the fluffy tip into the ear canal as far as it will go. The fluffy tip prevents the tip of the orange stick from damaging the eardrum, but be very careful not to push it into the ear canal too hard, and be prepared to let go of the mop if the patient jerks his head as you work it into the ear canal.

Work the mop out of the ear canal and inspect the fluffy tip to see what kind of discharge you have been able to clean out – usually purulent but sometimes discoloured by wax. Occasionally there will be some blood-staining. As long as you are not hurting the patient, there is no reason to stop mopping if there is blood-staining, but you should not continue to mop if there is blood-staining and mopping is painful. In this circumstance, consider syringing to clean the ear canal – see *Syringing of ears* below.

Take off the cotton wool, make another mop, and clean the ear canal again. Repeat this until no more discharge is being mopped out.

When the ear canal is dry, examine the ear with an otoscope. You want to check that you have managed to get all the discharge and debris cleaned out. If not, you can either continue mopping or resort to syringing – see *Syringing of ears* below. Once the canal is clean, examine both the ear canal and the eardrum to make a diagnosis.

If you lose the cotton wool part of the mop in the ear canal, you will have to get it out again. Try and catch it with a pair of fine-toothed forceps and remove it. If this is unsuccessful, you will have to try and syringe it out.

Once you are experienced with making mops and mopping patients' ears you can teach your patients, or the attending adult in the case of children, how to make up mops and how to clean their own ears.

Syringing of ears

Syringing is a way of cleaning out ear canals by flushing them with a gentle jet of water. The most important point to remember about syringing is that the temperature of the syringing water has to be exactly the same as body temperature. If it is either too hot or too cold, syringing is going to induce vertigo (remember the caloric test for vestibular function!), a sensation described as 'being drunk in the head'. This occurs because the balance organ in the inner ear is close to the ear canal and is easily upset by changes in temperature. Syringing is a safe technique to use, provided it is done gently and only for ears with either a foreign body, wax, purulent discharge, or infected debris in the ear canal. After syringing it is essential that you examine the ear canal to check that you have indeed cleaned it out and that you are now able to examine the eardrum.

To syringe ears you will need a suitable syringe. The usual one is large and made of metal with loops for your fingers; see Figure 14.3. One problem with this type of syringe is that the plunger is often tight and does not move up and down easily inside the barrel of the syringe. If this is the case, take the syringe apart and clean the plunger and the inside of the barrel. You may need to use wire wool, an abrasive scourer, or scouring powder to get the metal surfaces clean and shiny. Apply a coating of Vaseline® or something similarly greasy to both the plunger and the inside of the barrel and then try it again.

An alternative is to use the largest size of syringe that you can find, if at all possible one with finger loops because these syringes require only one hand for filling each time they are emptied. Do not use a metal needle but use either a suction catheter, which is then cut short, or a wide-bore intravenous cannula. It must fit onto the syringe tightly and not come off when you squirt a jet of water through it as hard as you can. Test it a few times to make sure of this before you use it but remember that you will only syringe an ear with a gentle squirt!

You will also need a jug or bowl for the syringing water, a bowl or receiver to catch the water as it pours out of the ear, and a towel or waterproof to keep the patient dry.

Syringing is done in good light so that you can see where you are placing the tip on the syringe. The patient should be sitting sideways-on in front of you with the ear to be syringed pointing towards the source of light. A child should be seated on an adult's lap with both the head and the body firmly held. Place the towel or the waterproof around the patient so that he will not get too wet. Older children and adults are shown how to hold the receiving container so that it catches the water that will come out of the ear. For co-operative younger children the attending adult should be able to hold the receiving container at the same time as holding the child but for less co-operative children a second assistant will have to be enrolled for this task.

Check the water temperature with the back of your hand – it should be exactly body temperature, no warmer and no colder. Fill and squirt out the syringe a few times to check that it is working smoothly. Fill the syringe and hold it in one hand. With the other hand gently pull the pinna of the external ear away from the head – this helps to straighten out the ear canal – and then place the tip on the syringe just next to or just into the ear canal and gently empty the syringe, directing the stream of water into the ear canal. Check the water that has come out into your receiving container to see what you have been able to flush out of the ear.

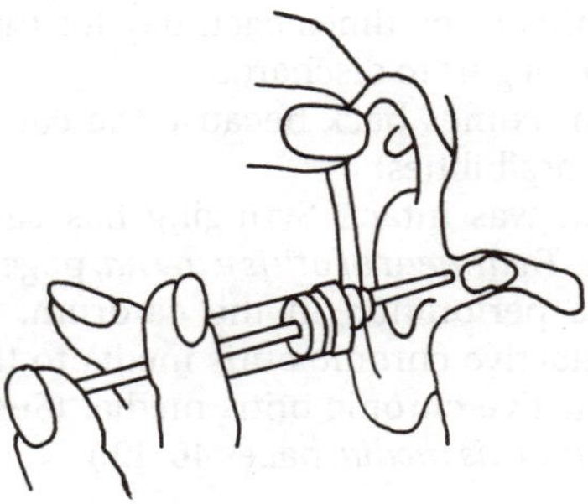

Figure 14.3 Ear syringing

Repeat this a few times and then examine the ear canal with your otoscope. Repeat the whole process a few times until the ear canal is clean.

It is sometimes difficult to get hard, impacted wax out of the ear canal. If this is the case, remember that wax dissolves in water. Lie the patient down with the wax-filled ear uppermost and fill the ear canal with water. Get the patient to pump it about a bit for ten minutes – refilling the canal a few times – and then try syringing again. Repeat this again if necessary. If this doesn't work, ask the patient to fill his ear with water and to pump it about a few times during the rest of the day and return the next day for another attempt.

When it is clean, examine the ear canal to check that you have not caused any injury by scratching it with the tip on the syringe. If you have scratched it, explain to the patient what has happened and put some ear drops in. Explain that he should return if the ear becomes sore or begins to discharge. If there is no injury, dry the ear canal by dry mopping (see above), and you will be able to examine the eardrum. If the problem for which you were syringing the ear was a discharge, you should now be able to see the eardrum well enough to make a diagnosis. If the problem was wax or a foreign body, you should check that there is not a perforation in the eardrum because, if there is a perforation, it is a possibility that the syringing may cause infection to flare up. To prevent this you should instill ear drops and instruct the patient to do this three times each day for two days and to return if the ear begins to discharge.

If the patient comes back because the ear is discharging there are two possibilities:

- The eardrum was intact. Syringing has caused an otitis externa. (See *Treatment of otitis externa*, pages 41-42.)
- There was a perforation in the eardrum. Syringing has caused an inactive chronic otitis media to flare up and to become an active chronic otitis media. (See *Treatment of active chronic otitis media*, pages 46-49.)

Instilling ear drops

Three different types of ear drops are used for treating ear infections. Ear drops may be antiseptic – an example is boracic ear drops, a cheap 'all round' preparation to use. They may be acidification agents – an example is 2 per cent acetic acid ear drops. These are used particularly for Pseudomonas infection – very common in active chronic otitis media. Lastly they may contain specific antibiotics. These latter drops tend to be expensive but are generally more effective than the others at clearing up infection. It is worth remembering that some ear drops burn or sting for a short while after they have been instilled and patients need to be warned about this. If you find that your patient will not use a particular ear drop because of this then try a different preparation.

When instilling an ear drop it should be obvious that the drop is not going to do any good unless it penetrates down to the area of infection. This will not be possible if the ear canal is full of pus or debris, so that cleaning of the ear canal is an essential first step (see *Dry mopping*, page 187, and *Syringing*, page 189). To successfully instill ear drops, the light needs to be good enough for you to see where the ear drops are being placed. The patient should lie on her side or tilt her head so that the ear into which the drop is to be instilled is pointing upwards. Gently pull the pinna away from the head to straighten the ear canal. Drop two or three drops directly into the ear canal – if you miss, wiggle the pinna about until the drops run into the canal. Once the ear drops are in the ear canal, wiggle the pinna about until the drops run all the way down to the bottom of the canal and drop in a further two or three drops. Then place a finger on the tragus – the small bump just in front of the ear canal – and squash it down so that it closes off the canal. Repeat this pumping action a few times. This helps to spread the ear drops around inside the ear canal and also pushes some of the drops through into the middle ear if there is a perforation in the eardrum. (Sometimes the drops go all the way down the eustachian tube and the patient can then taste them!) The patient should stay on her side for a further minute. As she straightens her head, some of the drops may run out and need to be wiped away.

This technique should be taught to the person who will be going to instill the ear drops at home. It is difficult for patients to instill ear drops into their own ears but if they do not have anyone to do it for them they will have to learn how to do it as well as they can.

Removal of a foreign body from the nose

These patients will usually be small, unco-operative children whose parents will either have noticed or been told about the foreign body or noted a unilateral, often foul-smelling, discharge from the nose. Parents will often have tried to get the child to blow it out but if they haven't, and the child will co-operate, this is worth trying initially.

Wrap the child up in a sheet and sit him upright, facing you, on the parent's lap with the child's legs restrained by the parent's crossed legs, one of the parent's arms holding the child's body and the other firmly holding the child's head. See Figure 14.4.

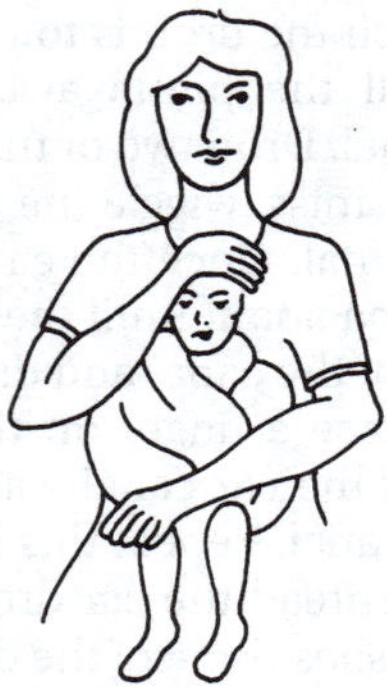

Figure 14.4 Wrapping up and holding a child for nasal procedure

Confirm the presence of the foreign body, using a head light, if available, a torch, or an otoscope with a large speculum. You may need to suction away any accumulated secretions to see it. Is it a solid object or something soft such as sponge or paper? If something soft it can usually be grasped with a fine-toothed forceps and removed. If it is solid do not attempt to grasp it as it may slide deeper into the nasal cavity.

For solid objects, take a probe with a curved tip in one hand, steady the nose with the other hand, and pass the tip of the probe along the floor of the nose until it is past the object. Elevate the tip, trapping the object between the probe and the dorsum of the nasal cavity. Keeping the tip elevated, draw the probe out of the nose, bringing the foreign body with it until it reaches the vestibule when it can be extruded by pinching behind it with the thumb and first finger of the hand on the nose. The nose may bleed a little, especially if there is an infection, but this will soon stop. See Figure 14.5.

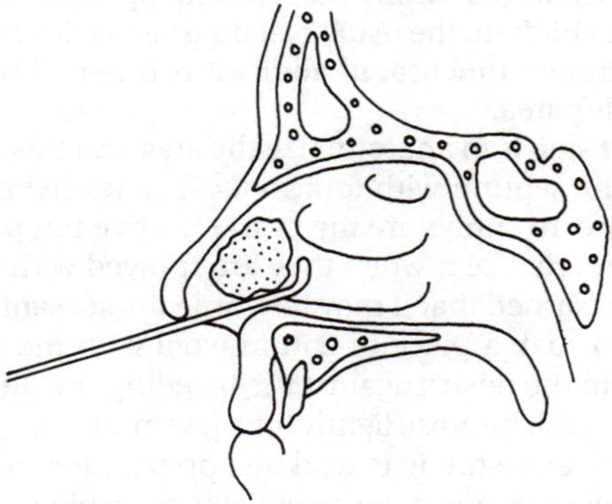

Figure 14.5 Removing a foreign body from the nose

If unsuccessful, re-examine the nose and if the foreign body is still visible, try again. If still unsuccessful it is worth a third attempt before resorting to either a general anaesthetic or, if available, referral to a specialist service.

Cauterizing a nose

Patients suitable for cautery will be those with a bleeding site that is visible and accessible on the anterior nasal septum.

Active bleeding will need to be controlled before attempting cautery. Soak a piece of cotton wool in some vasoconstrictor nasal drops, place this into the nostril to rest against the bleeding site and request the patient to pinch his nose for five to ten minutes. Then gently remove the cotton wool.

The first step in cautery is to accurately identify the bleeding site. If a headlight is available, gently insert a nasal speculum into the nostril to open it out and push the hairs out of the way, then inspect the anterior septum. If not, many otoscopes are supplied with a fat nasal speculum which is very useful in adults. In children, you will have to use the largest ear speculum – which is too small to cauterize through, but children don't have hairy noses and the area can often be seen by just tilting the nasal tip upwards a little with a finger. In children, the usual bleeding vessel lies at the junction of skin and mucosa, in adults it is often a little behind this in Little's area.

The next step is to anaesthetize the area and this is done by spraying the septum with topical local anaesthetic solution. The 10 per cent sprays are the most effective but patients do not particularly like it when they are sprayed with them and need to be warned that it may be a little unpleasant. An alternative is to soak a piece of cotton wool with the spray and place this in the nostril against the bleeding site. Request the patient to pinch his nose lightly for a few minutes.

While the anaesthetic is working, prepare for cautery. The most useful device is a commercially available orange stick tipped with solid silver nitrate. Also prepare two or three orange sticks with cotton wool tips – these will be used to apply pressure should the bleeding point start bleeding when the silver nitrate is applied to it. Make two or three small balls of cotton wool for placing in the nostril and have a pair of forceps handy for manipulating them.

Once the mucosa is anaesthetized, reposition the speculum so that you can see the bleeding point and then touch this lightly with the stick tipped with silver nitrate. The mucosa will turn white as the silver nitrate burns it. Cauterize the bleeding point but as little of the mucosa around it as possible.

If it starts bleeding, take one of the sticks tipped with cotton wool and apply pressure to the bleeding point for a minute. Repeat the cautery as the blood may have washed the silver nitrate away before it effectively cauterized the vessel.

Place a piece of cotton wool in the nostril and leave it there for ten minutes. Silver nitrate stains the skin black and doing this prevents nasal secretions contaminated with silver nitrate from running out onto the skin. It is also useful to coat the skin with Vaseline® before beginning to cauterize in order to prevent staining.

Warn the patient that a small scab will form and there may

be bleeding if the scab is dislodged but that this should be easily controlled by pinching the nose. Advise the patient to apply a little Vaseline® or antiseptic cream to the cauterized area for a few days. Healing should be complete in about ten days.

Draining a quinsy

Quinsy is the term used to describe an abscess that develops in severe tonsillitis between the affected tonsil and its bed between the two pillars of the fauces. It is an intensely painful condition. The patients (usually young adults or older children) are toxic, cannot swallow, and often the inflammation has caused spasm of the masticatory muscles so that they have trismus as well. If a view can be obtained, the soft palate on the affected side will be seen to be inflamed and swollen and the tonsil to be pushed across to the midline.

It is a very satisfying condition to treat as relief of the intense pain is almost instantaneous if the pus can be drained – although patients still have a very sore throat for several days afterwards! If they can open their mouth sufficiently, treatment is accomplished either by aspiration or by incision. If not, you will have to refer them as an emergency to have this done under a general anaesthetic. If an anaesthetic is needed many practitioners will opt to do a 'hot' tonsillectomy to avoid having the patient come back to have the tonsils removed subsequently.

Spray the area well with 10 per cent topical local anaesthetic. While this is working, prepare either a syringe with a wide-bore needle or a scalpel. For the latter use a No. 11 blade – long and pointed – and wrap strapping around the blade so that only 1 cm of the tip is exposed – this prevents inadvertent deep penetration. You will need a receiver for the patient to spit into, a mug with mouthwash and a spatula – if available, a metal tongue spatula.

Depress the tongue and select a point at the junction of imaginary lines running vertically up the anterior pillar and horizontally at the junction of uvula with soft palate. If

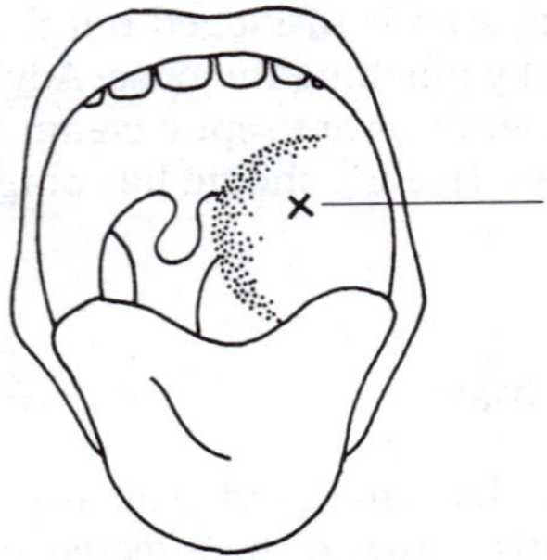

Figure 14.6 Draining or aspirating a quinsy

aspirating, penetrate at this point to a depth of about 1 cm and aspirate the pus. If incising, do the same with the scalpel blade and let the pus pour out to be spat into the receiver. See Figure 14.6.

If no pus is obtained, either the quinsy was not 'ripe' or you have not penetrated deeply enough. If the patient will allow you to do so, try again.

Whether you obtain pus or not, these patients require emergency admission as they need not only analgesics but IV antibiotic and fluids until they can swallow again. Thereafter antibiotic is continued until the tonsillitis has settled and a few weeks later the tonsils should be removed.

Emergency aspiration of a retropharyngeal abscess in an infant

A retropharyngeal abscess is diagnosed from a lateral neck X-ray and by palpation of the back of the throat with a finger tip. Normally it will be drained under the controlled conditions afforded by a general anaesthetic. Sometimes, however, the diagnosis is missed in infants until they present with severe upper airway obstruction. This can be an emergency situation. When a laryngoscope is inserted to see what is causing the obstruction, a large swelling will be seen to be obstructing the back of the pharynx.

Prepare a syringe with a wide-bore needle and a suction apparatus with a suitable throat suction nozzle (not a suction catheter). Wrap the infant in a sheet and lie him on his back with the head extended and some support under his shoulders. If possible, the table should be tilted so that the patient is in a head-down position. Insert the laryngoscope, penetrate the abscess with the needle, and aspirate as much of the pus as possible. Immediately turn the infant onto his side and suction the back of the throat for as long as pus continues to drain.

This should restore the airway and allow time to make arrangements for emergency admission.

Securing an emergency airway

Most resuscitation first aid kits will contain a laryngoscope and a selection of endotracheal tubes. This is the preferred method of securing an airway when positioning the patient or insertion of an oral airway has not proven adequate. If time permits, try to spray the back of the throat with topical anaesthetic before attempting to pass the laryngoscope as this will reduce the amount of gagging. Give another spray to the larynx as soon as it is visible to reduce the tendency for laryngospasm before attempting to pass the tube.

Although intubation is usually feasible, you will encounter emergency situations in which it may not be possible to either see the larynx or pass an endotracheal tube. Quite often obstructed patients, who are dying, vomit, usually as a response to your attempt to pass the laryngoscope. Unless a suction apparatus is available that can cope with large volumes of partially digested food you are going to find it impossible to see the larynx and inhalation of gastric content almost always occurs in this situation. For this reason always ask someone to apply very firm 'cricoid pressure' before attempting to pass the laryngoscope.

Severe head and neck trauma also presents a difficult situation because displaced skeletal elements and copious bleeding often make intubation an impossible task. In this situation, if the patient is unconscious, try positioning and insertion of an oral airway before considering intubation. A conscious patient will not tolerate an oral airway and an alternative is to try and pass as large an endotracheal tube as will fit through the nose into the pharynx to act as an airway.

If all else fails and the situation is desperate, you will have to resort to methods of desperation. The first of these is the cricothyrotomy; see Figure 14.7. Position the patient on her back with the head extended and if possible something under the shoulders. This brings the larynx and trachea forwards into prominence. Identify the cricothyroid membrane which lies between the lower border of the thyroid cartilage and the cricoid, which is the uppermost and most prominent of the tracheal rings. At its simplest, cricothyrotomy involves placing wide-bore needles through this membrane into the trachea, connecting these to a source of oxygen and blowing oxygen into the trachea in as large a volume as the system will permit. If these are not available you will have to resort to taking a scalpel, plunging it horizontally through the membrane – it will bleed a lot – and then twisting the blade vertically to open the space created. A small uncuffed endotracheal tube can then be passed through this opening into the trachea.

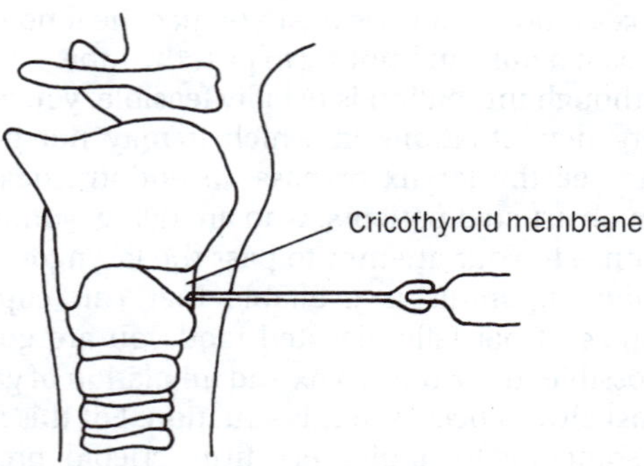

Figure 14.7 Emergency cricothyrotomy

An alternative to the cricothyrotomy is to undertake an emergency tracheostomy. Position the patient as above.

Prepare a narrow, cuffed endotracheal tube. Grasp the trachea firmly between the thumb and first finger midway between the cricoid and the sternal notch, stretching the skin tightly over it. Take a scalpel in the other hand, take a deep breath and, with a single, deep, vertical incision, cut into the midline of the trachea. It will bleed a lot but immediately pass the endotracheal tube and inflate the cuff. Draw back the tube until the cuff lies just below your incision, otherwise the end of the tube will be lying in the right main bronchus, pack the wound with a gauze dressing and secure the tube.

Glossary

This glossary contains some of the terminology generally used by tutors and others in an ENT department and in this manual.

Acoustic neuroma. A benign tumour (schwannoma) arising on either the auditory or the vestibular portions of the 8th cranial nerve.
Anosmia. A loss of the sense of smell.
Antrostomy. Procedure to form an opening from the nasal cavity into the maxillary sinus (maxillary antrum). The opening may be made in either the inferior or the middle meatus.
Antrum washout. Irrigation of the maxillary sinus after placing a trocar and cannula into the sinus from beneath the inferior turbinate. Used to determine the presence of pus in the sinus and to wash out inspissated pus.
Aphonia. Loss of the voice.
Aphthous ulcers. Ulceration of the oral mucosa of unknown aetiology.
Atrophic rhinitis. See Ozaena.
Atticotomy. A surgical procedure to expose the attic area of the middle ear cavity.
Audiometry. A method of testing the hearing using an audiometer, a machine producing pure tones which can be varied in frequency and intensity.

Barotrauma. A disorder resulting from acute pressure change such as may occur in diving or flying. Acute negative pressure change in the middle ear causes an effusion, whereas acute positive pressure change can result in round window rupture (inner ear fistula).
Bell's palsy (Syn. idiopathic facial nerve palsy). A neuritis of the 7th cranial nerve of unknown aetiology.
Blow-out fracture. A fracture of the floor of the orbit resulting from the acute pressure increase of a direct blow to the globe. Orbital contents are extruded into and trapped in the fracture, resulting in limitation of globe movement.
Branchial cyst. A cystic swelling originating from embryological remnants retained in the lines of fusion of the branchial clefts.

Caldwell-Luc antrostomy. A surgical approach into the maxillary sinus through a sublabial incision. The anterior wall of the sinus is removed to expose the sinus contents.
Caloric test. Stimulation of the vestibular system to produce

nystagmus by irrigating the ear canal with water either above or below body temperature. The amount of stimulation is monitored with an electronystagmogram (ENG).

Choanae. The posterior openings of the nasal cavities into the nasopharynx.

Cholesteatoma. Disease of the middle ear that starts when a retraction pocket forms in the eardrum in response to negative middle ear pressure. Since the outside layer of the drum is squamous epithelium, this now forms the lining of the pocket. These pockets behave rather like epidermoid cysts and invade the middle ear cleft.

Chorda tympani nerve. A branch of the facial nerve that crosses the middle ear cavity. It carries efferent secretomotor fibres to the submandibular and sublingual salivary glands and afferent taste fibres from the anterior two-thirds of the tongue.

Cochlea. The coiled auditory receptor organ of the inner ear.

Commando procedure. A surgical procedure for ablating malignant disease of the floor of the mouth/tonsil area. It involves extensive resection of the floor of the mouth, pharynx, and mandible, combined with a radical neck dissection of all lymph node containing tissue. Flaps containing skin, muscle, and sometimes bone are needed for reconstruction.

Conductive deafness. Loss of hearing resulting from disorders in the external and middle ears. Distinguished clinically from sensorineural deafness by use of a tuning fork.

Cribriform plate. The thin plate of bone separating the roof of the nose from the anterior cranial fossa. It is perforated by the olfactory nerve fibres.

Croup. A popular term for laryngo-tracheo-bronchitis (LTB) that describes the typical cough.

Dysphagia. Difficulty in swallowing. When swallowing is painful it is known as odynophagia.

Dysphonia. A weakness of the voice rather than a hoarseness, caused either by recurrent laryngeal nerve palsy or a functional disorder.

Endolymphatic hydrops (Syn. Ménières disease). Refers to the increase in pressure that occurs in the endolymphatic duct of the cochlea, precipitating the symptoms of tinnitus, vertigo, and deafness.

Epiglottitis (Syn. supraglottitis). An acute bacterial infection of the supraglottic mucosa of the larynx. Inflammatory swelling rapidly causes total airway obstruction.

Epiphora. Tears spilling over the eyelid rather than draining down the nasolacrimal duct.

Epistaxis. Bleeding from the nose.

Erythroplakia. An area of mucosal dysplasia without hyperkeratosis, hence having a red appearance rather than the white appearance of leukoplakia. May be a premalignant lesion.
Ethmoidal sinuses. A group of small air cells situated between the upper nasal cavity and the orbit.
Exostosis. A bony growth in the deep portion of the external ear canal. Seen most frequently in people who swim in cold water.

Facial nerve. The 7th cranial nerve. Intimately related to the inner and middle ear in its passage through the temporal bone.
Frontal sinus trephine. A drainage procedure for the frontal sinus performed through a skin incision above the medial canthus of the eye.
Fronto-ethmoidectomy. A surgical procedure to eradicate disease from the frontal and ethmoidal sinuses during which a wide drainage pathway is created into the nasal cavity. The surgery may be performed either internally using nasal endoscopy instrumentation, or externally through a Lynch incision around the medial canthus of the eye.
Furuncle. A localized abscess (boil) arising in a hair follicle. In ENT, these abscesses are seen in the hair-bearing skin of the external ear canal or in the nasal vestibule.

Glandular fever (Syn. infectious mononucleosis). A severe tonsillitis with sloughing of the surface mucosa and a marked lymphadenopathy. There may be associated hepatosplenomegaly.
Globus syndrome. A term used to describe the sensation of a lump in the throat when there is no discernible organic cause.
Glomus tumour. A tumour arising from chemoreceptor cells. In ENT, these tumours are seen either in the middle ear (glomus tympanicum) or arising from the jugular bulb (glomus jugulare).
Glossopharyngeal nerve. The 9th cranial nerve supplying sensation to much of the pharynx.
Glottis. The anatomical area of the true vocal cords in the larynx. The supraglottis is the area of the larynx above the cords. The subglottis is the area of the larynx below the cords.
Glue ear (Syn. otitis media with effusion). Refers to the thick, tenacious mucus found in the middle ear in this disorder.
Goitre. A generalized enlargement of the thyroid gland.
Grommet. A minute ventilation tube placed in the tympanic membrane to aerate the middle ear in otitis media with effusion, a disorder arising from eustachian tube dysfunction.

Haemotympanum. The presence of blood within the middle

ear that imparts a bruised discoloration to the tympanic membrane.

Hallpike's test. A manoeuvre to test for the presence of positional vertigo.

Heimlich's manoeuvre. A manoeuvre to attempt to dislodge an impacted foreign body obstructing the airway by placing the arms around the patient from behind and applying sharp, forcible pressure to the upper abdomen and diaphragm.

Hoarseness. A change in the voice from normal to having a rough quality.

Hypoglossal nerve. The 12th cranial nerve that supplies motor efferent fibres to the muscles of the tongue.

Hypopharynx. The inferior portion of the pharynx. The larynx forms its anterior wall. The areas on either side of the larynx are known as the pyriform fossae. The area between these, behind the larynx, is known as the postcricoid region. The hypopharynx opens inferiorly into the upper oesophagus through the cricopharyngeal sphincter.

Idiopathic facial nerve palsy. See Bell's palsy.

Impedence audiometry. See Tympanometry.

Infectious mononucleosis. See Glandular fever.

Labyrinth. The complex of spaces and canals that comprise the inner ear, consisting of the cochlea and vestibular system. Labyrinthitis refers to infection. Labyrinthectomy refers to a destructive surgical procedure.

Laryngectomy. A surgical procedure for malignant disease of the larynx involving removal of all or a portion of the larynx.

Laryngitis. Inflammation of the laryngeal mucosa. In infancy this is usually part of a more generalized laryngo-tracheo-bronchitis (LTB or croup).

Laryngoscopy. Examination of the larynx. Indirect laryngoscopy is performed with a mirror. Direct laryngoscopy is performed with a flexible fibre-optic endoscope while the patient is awake or with a laryngoscope while the patient is under anaesthetic.

Laryngo-tracheo-bronchitis (LTB). See Croup.

Le Fort fractures. Fractures of the facial skeleton.

Leukoplakia (cf. erythroplakia). An area of mucosal dysplasia with hyperkeratosis giving it a white appearance. May be a premalignant lesion.

Little's area. An area of prominent vasculature on the anterior nasal septum.

Ludwig's angina. Infection of the floor of the mouth and submental tissues, usually arising from dental infection. Swelling can push the tongue upwards and backwards to cause upper airway obstruction.

Mastoidectomy. A surgical procedure to eradicate mastoid disease. Cortical mastoidectomy refers to exenteration of all the mastoid air cells, the resulting cavity draining into the middle ear. Radical mastoidectomy refers to extending this by removal of the posterior wall of the ear canal so that the resulting cavity opens into the ear canal.
Ménières disease. See Endolymphatic hydrops.
Mesotympanum. The middle ear cavity.
Myringitis. Inflammation of the tympanic membrane.
Myringoplasty. Surgical grafting of a defect in the tympanic membrane.
Myringotomy. An incision into the tympanic membrane that is usually followed by insertion of a grommet tube.

Nasopharynx (Syn. postnasal space). That portion of the pharynx above the soft palate containing the adenoid and the eustachian cushions (the openings of the eustachian tubes). The fossa of Rosenmüller lies between the eustachian cushion and the choana.
Neck dissection (Syn. block dissection, radical neck dissection). Surgical excision of all tissue containing lymph nodes from the neck undertaken to eradicate metastatic malignant disease.
Neuropraxia. A temporary block to nerve conduction.
Nystagmus. The physical sign indicating a vestibular disorder in which the eyes slowly drift laterally and then quickly revert centrally. The nystagmus is named in the direction of the quick component. See Vestibulo-ocular reflex.

Obstructive apnoea. Inspiratory efforts are unable to overcome upper airway obstruction so that there is no air flow into the lungs. When severe, the condition is known as obstructive sleep apnoea syndrome, which has complications and can precipitate cardiac failure.
Odynophagia. Painful dysphagia.
Oro-antral fistula. A persistent opening from the maxillary sinus into the oral cavity that usually follows extraction of infected upper teeth whose roots project into the floor of the sinus.
Ossiculoplasty. Surgical reconstruction of a sound-conducting mechanism in the middle ear using either ossicle remnants or a prosthesis.
Ostium. The natural opening of a sinus into the nasal cavity. Most open beneath the middle turbinate into the middle meatus, an area known as the ostiomeatal complex.
Otalgia. Pain in the ear due either to local ear disease or referred from other sites.
Otitis media with effusion. See

Glue ear.
Otomycosis. Fungal otitis externa.
Otorrhoea. Discharge from the ear.
Otosclerosis. A disorder in which the stapes becomes fixed in the oval window by localized, abnormal bony overgrowth to cause a conduction deafness.
Ototoxicity. Damage to hair cells of either the cochlea or vestibular system as a side-effect of some drugs.
Ozaena (Syn. atrophic rhinitis). Refers to the smell of chronic infection related to the crusting that occurs in the nasal cavity in this condition.

Pansinusitis. Infection involving all of the sinuses.
Perilymph. The fluid in the inner ear perilymphatic compartment surrounding the endolymphatic compartment (which contains the hair cells).
Pharyngeal pouch. A herniation through the inferior constrictor muscle of the pharynx.
Postnasal space. See Nasopharynx.
Presbyacusis. The sensorineural deafness of ageing that results from gradual loss of hair cells and predominantly affects the higher tones.

Quinsy. An abscess that forms in the bed of the tonsil during a severe tonsillitis.

Ranula. A cystic swelling in the floor of the mouth that results from obstruction of the duct of a mucus-secreting gland.
Reinke's oedema. Oedematous swelling in the submucosa of the vocal cords (Reinke's space).
Rhinoplasty. An operation to alter the external appearance of the nose.
Rhinorrhoea. Discharge from the nose.
Rinne's test. A tuning fork test to distinguish between conduction and sensorineural deafness.
Romberg's test. A test to determine an individual's ability to maintain balance when standing with the eyes closed.

Sensorineural deafness. Deafness due to causes within the inner ear and/or its neural pathway.
Septoplasty. An operation to straighten a deviated nasal septum, preserving the septal cartilage (cf. submucous resection).
Sialectasis. Dilatation of the ducts in a salivary gland distal to obstruction of minor ducts within the gland.
Sicca syndrome. See Sjögren's syndrome.
Sjögren's syndrome (Syn. sicca syndrome). An auto-immune disorder affecting exocrine glands. In ENT, the effects seen include decreased lacrimation, dryness of the mucous membranes in the nose and mouth, and swelling of the parotid glands.

Speech audiometry. A method of assessing hearing using spoken words in place of pure tones through an audiometer.
Stapedectomy. A surgical procedure in which the fixed stapes due to otosclerosis is replaced with a prosthesis.
Stapedius reflex. The reflex contraction of the stapedius muscle in the middle ear in response to loud sounds. This movement can be detected using a tympanometer.
Stridor. The high-pitched sound produced by obstruction in the airway in either the larynx (inspiratory) or the trachea (expiratory).
Submucous resection (SMR). An operation to straighten a deviated nasal septum involving removal of septal cartilage.
Supraglottitis. See Epiglottitis.

Thyroglossal cyst. A cystic swelling of embryological remnants left in the line of descent of the thyroid gland.
Tinnitus. Stimulation of the auditory system by something other than external sounds.
Tonsils. The collection of lymphoid tissue situated between the anterior and posterior 'pillars' at the entrance to the pharynx. They form part of Waldeyer's ring of lymphoid tissue around the upper aerodigestive tract.
Tracheostomy. A surgical procedure to create an opening from the anterior neck into the trachea for both respiration and aspiration of secretions.
Tympanometry (Syn. impedance audiometry). A method of assessing the status of the tympanic membrane (tympanogram), the middle ear pressure, and the 'stapedius reflex' using an instrument known as a tympanometer.
Tympanoplasty. A surgical procedure to reconstruct both the tympanic membrane (myringoplasty) and the ossicular chain (ossiculoplasty).
Tympanosclerosis. Calcified scarring of the tympanic membrane often seen after grommet insertion.
Tympanotomy. A surgical procedure to elevate the tympanic membrane in order to examine the middle ear.

Uvulo-palato-pharyngoplasty (UV3P). A surgical procedure to tighten up the soft palate to prevent snoring.

Valsalva manoeuvre. By pinching the nose shut, holding the mouth closed, and blowing hard the pressure generated can inflate the middle ear.
Vasomotor rhinitis. One form of non-allergic rhinitis characterized by persistent swelling of the mucosa over the inferior turbinates thought to be due to parasympathetic overactivity.
Vertebro-basilar insufficiency. Temporary interruption of blood flow in the vertebral

artery when pinched by movements of the arthritic cervical spine. Causes 'drop attacks' and may precipitate vertigo.
Vertigo. The sensation of rotatory movement caused by vestibular system disorders.
Vestibular neuronitis. One of the causes of vertigo due to a neuritis affecting the vestibular nerve; of unknown aetiology.
Vestibulo-ocular reflex. The mechanism whereby an image stays focused on one portion of the retina during movement of the head.

Index